Critical Care Nursing

Studies in Health, Illness, and Caregiving

Joan E. Lynaugh, Series Editor

A complete list of books in the series is available from the publisher.

Critical Care Nursing

A History

Julie Fairman and Joan E. Lynaugh

with a Foreword by Gladys M. Campbell and Barbara Siebelt

PENN

University of Pennsylvania Press

Philadelphia

10 9 8 7 6 5 4 3 2 1

Published by
University of Pennsylvania Press
Philadelphia, Pennsylvania 19104-4011

Library of Congress Cataloging-in-Publication Data
Fairman, Julie.
    Critical care nursing : a history / Julie Fairman and Joan E. Lynaugh.
       p.   cm. — (Studies in health, illness, and caregiving)
    Includes bibliographical references and index.
    ISBN 0-8122-3258-5 (alk. paper)
    1. Intensive care nursing—History. I. Lynaugh, Joan E. II. Title. III. Series.
    [DNLM: 1. History of Nursing—United States.   2. Critical Care—history—
United States.   WY 11 F17c 1998]
RT120.I5F34   1998
610.73′61—dc21
DNLM/DLC
for Library of Congress   97-50184
                                                                            CIP

Contents

Foreword

Critical care nurses have always cared for the most vulnerable patients and their families. Over the past decades the healthcare environment has changed dramatically, yet our values and the focus of our practice have remained constant. We have continued to center our practice on patients and families. This focus and the potential for unsafe patient care situations led early nurse and physician reformers collaboratively to challenge traditional hospital nursing and healthcare systems. In telling our history, we remember the origins of our practice and see the connection with our past, present, and future through the continuity of our vision and principles. Although not published until 1992, AACN's vision of a healthcare system driven by the needs of patients and their families, in which critical care nurses make their optimal contribution, has been actualized through our shared values throughout our history.

From the beginnings of our practice in the 1960s, the founders of critical care nursing and of AACN valued and fought for humane, effective, collaborative, and accessible care for the nation's critically ill citizens. These firsthand accounts, told by an earlier generation of nurses who changed the way patients were cared for in hospitals, remind us that it is like-minded individuals banding together who improve and sustain society. In 1969, nurses imagined AACN as an inclusive organization committed to investigation, education, and communication about caring for the critically ill. That is precisely the organization we know today. Although much larger and more influential, the AACN of today remains steadfast in its values and principles. As in the past, it is through our association with each other and our united commitment to a vision of a patient-centered healthcare system that we find the inspiration and strength to deliver excellence in caring for critically ill patients and their families and ensure opportunities for nurses to make their optimal contribution. This is the firm foundation on which we will build a better future for healthcare. We hope this history provides insight, confidence, courage, and commitment as today's critical care nurses extend the vision and the values of those who went before us to the patients we care for today.

Gladys M. Campbell, RN, MSN
President, AACN
1997–1998

Barbara Siebelt, RN, BA
President, AACN
1969–1970

Acknowledgments

Over the years we worked on this study, we have appreciated the support and advice of all our colleagues and friends. For research funding we are very grateful to the American Association of Critical-Care Nurses, which sponsored the study. Additional research support came from the American Nurses' Foundation and the American Organization of Nurse Executives. Julie Fairman also received a postdoctoral fellowship from the Center for the Study of the History of Nursing, School of Nursing, University of Pennsylvania.

We are especially grateful to scholars at the history center for their commentary on and critique of the various papers and presentations leading up to this book. In particular, we would like to thank members of the "round table," including Karen Buhler-Wilkerson, Ellen Baer, Patricia D'Antonio, Barbara Brush, and Janna Dieckmann. Historians Rosemary Stevens and Judith McGaw offered both early guidance and a framework for thinking about this complicated story. Mary Norris read the entire manuscript and offered invaluable editorial criticism and suggestions.

This book could never have been written without the insights and poignant stories of the more than seventy critical care nurses, physicians, and administrators we interviewed. We wish to especially thank the staffs of Chestnut Hill Hospital (CHH) in Chestnut Hill, Pennsylvania, and Hospital of the University of Pennsylvania (HUP) in Philadelphia for their interest and the time they took to talk with us. We thank the officers and staff of the American Association of Critical-Care Nurses, who were generous with their own irreplaceable experiences, and who gave us free access to their archives. The staff at CHH and those holding the valuable records of HUP proved indispensable to our project. In particular, Nadine Landis had the foresight to rescue and preserve the nursing records at HUP. Susan Mowery, the former medical librarian at CHH, also deserves special thanks.

Last, we thank our families and friends. In particular, Ron, Alex, and Connor deserve much more than thanks for their understanding, support, and patience during the last several years it took to bring this project to fruition.

Chapter 1
Inventing Critical Care Nursing

During the 1950s, 1960s, and 1970s, the essential elements of patient needs, growing medical knowledge, increased governmental funding, and changing societal values came together to stimulate a radical and sometimes chaotic reorganization of nursing care in hospitals. The now ubiquitous intensive care units grew out of a combination of professional interest in change and new public expectations for care. Although opposition arose from some, critical care was enthusiastically embraced by most professionals and the public, who at the time shared a simple understanding of the drive to preserve human life—seeing almost all interventions as an unalloyed good.[1]

Now, after forty years of experimentation, we are reevaluating our health care system and the moral and ethical implications of the accomplishments of critical care. What factors will influence how nurses respond to patients at risk and how will physically unstable patients at risk be protected? Where will this care occur? Who will be eligible to receive highly expensive, individualized "watchful vigilance"? Who will provide the care? This historical account is offered in the hope that it will help inform these debates.

Treating critical care nursing as a case study, we analyze the decision-making of hospitals and health care professionals concerning the changing needs of the patients they serve. We explore how intensive care units, one of the most obvious examples of post–World War II hospital reorganization, came to be; what goes on in these units; and how medical and nursing care of people in hospitals changed after critical care became established as a new, formalized category of patient care.

We explore the details of the origins of critical care, examining such questions as: How did critical care acquire its present form and importance? What forces stimulated this stunningly large investment in people, space, and technology? Who were the first critical care givers? Understanding the social, economic, scientific, and professional contributions that yielded this extremely popular, indeed dominant, aspect of hospital care helps explain both the sources and impetus for contemporary concerns.

To answer these questions we rely on the methods of social history, seeking to understand the reorganization of nursing and medical care in hospitals from the participants' standpoint. In particular we hope to place the now very large specialty of critical care nursing in historical context to better grasp the significance of its development. This account depends on the historical evidence left by nurses who, during the 1950s, 1960s, and 1970s, adapted their practice and became critical care nurses. We include the stories of physicians and hospital administrators, as well as organizational documents.

More than forty years ago, gathering critically ill patients together in intensive care units attracted controversy even as it became an extremely popular reform in hospital care. For example, when Dr. William McClenahan proposed to set aside a space for the concentrated nursing care of critically ill patients in 1953, the board of managers at Chestnut Hill Hospital (CHH) in Chestnut Hill, Pennsylvania, was reluctant to cooperate. Board members worried, quite predictably, about the expense; just as troubling to them was the idea of placing men and women in the same room. Only when McClenahan assured the board members that the patients would be too sick to care that the wards were mixed-sex did they go along with the proposal.[2]

Despite such worries at the outset, the use and growth of intensive care at CHH and others exceeded all expectations. When the American Hospital Association (AHA) began to collect statistics on intensive care units in 1959, there were just 238 units in short-term, voluntary, nonprofit hospitals.[3] By 1965, the AHA found 1,040 intensive care units, and in just six years, more than 90 percent of hospitals with 500 or more beds and 31 percent of those with 100 to 199 beds had opened intensive care units.[4]

Beginning just after World War II, the process of intensifying and improving nursing and medical care for some of the hospitals' sickest patients fascinated and consumed the resources of hospital leaders, nurses, and physicians. Critical care would prove to be a compelling, unsettling, much desired, and very expensive proposition in the history of American health care.

"Critical Care"

The phrase "critical care" is rather modern, but its meaning is quite old. Necessary to the current idea of critical care are two somewhat competitive constructs. The person who needs critical care must be physiologically unstable, at risk, or in danger of dying. On the other hand, intensive care is usually given to the person in the expectation or hope (however slim) of recovery. Thus, by definition, critical care melds physiological instability with hope for survival. To understand changes in critical care over time, it is important to bear in mind the prevailing definition of physiological instability, and the caregivers' expectation of positive results.

It is also important to recall that critically ill patients traditionally were protected by caregivers using two very consistent methods. First, caregivers "kept watch" by intensive observation; the ideal model of one nurse watching one patient was practiced by private-duty nurses. The second traditional way to protect the ill was patient triage, the sorting, grouping, and spatial arrangement of patients in proximity to the caregiver according to the stability of the patient's condition. Consider, for example, Louisa May Alcott's 1863 description of her nursing work after the battle at Fredericksburg, Virginia:

My ward is now divided into three rooms. . . . I had managed to sort out the patients in such a way that I had what I called "my duty room, my pleasure room, and my pathetic room," and worked for each in a different way. One I visited armed with a dressing tray full of rollers, plasters, and pins; another with books, flowers, games, and gossip; the third with teapots, lullabies, consolation, and, sometimes, a shroud . . . wherever the sickest or most helpless man chanced to be, there I held my watch.[5]

Alcott's poignant recollections show us that the practice of sorting the sick according to both intensity of needs and expectation of the outcome of illness coincided with that of gathering the sickest patients together so they could be observed more easily. Although Alcott could do little to cure her physically unstable patients, the ability to see and finally to comfort her patients justified her organization of care.

Similarly, Florence Nightingale advocated placing patients recovering from an operation or those needing large amounts of nursing care close to the nurses' desk, moving those requiring less care to the end of a ward or a quiet corner.[6] A twentieth-century nurse contributed this more recent description of her attempts to protect critically ill patients: "When I was first a nursing student I moved patients many times in the middle of the night in the ward. We kept our more acutely ill patients closest to the station. . . . You'd lose a patient so you'd bring your next most critical out."[7]

Changes in the hospital environment, such as staffing shortages or architectural modifications, could make traditional ministrations of care less effective, placing the critically ill patient at risk. For example, in one hospital in the early 1950s a seemingly physically stable four-year-old patient, alone in a private room at the end of the hall during a time of severe nursing shortage, experienced respiratory distress. She was saved only when a nurse happened to pass her room and recognize the child's danger.[8]

Available knowledge and useful drugs or treatments also influence the intensity and the actual work of caring for the critically ill. Consider the radical change in the concept of care for premature infants. In 1950, newborn babies of less than four pounds were put in incubators and merely observed. In the 1990s, the knowledge and technology exist to ventilate and nourish far tinier infants in the expectation that many will survive. Looking at the other end of life, an enormously wide and complex array of pharmacological and surgical interventions are now used to care for persons who suffer from advanced heart disease. The current expectation of changing the course of heart disease through therapeutic intervention is in sharp contrast to the goals of the simple bed rest and diuretic regimen prescribed for such patients forty years ago.

Changing Patterns of Patient Care and Public Expectations

The idea of gathering sick people together to provide safe, efficient, and humane care is the fundamental concept underlying the hospital and the impetus for the creation of nursing as paid work. In the creation of intensive care units and the field of critical care, however, there is a radical accentuation of the idea of gathering together the sickest patients—an approach emphasizing group care and putting expertise and efficiency above all else.

What was it about the 1950s and 1960s that inspired this extensive reorganization of care in hospitals—that is, the invention of critical care? Part of the explanation is found in the advent of an increasingly complex hospital population for whom, at last, more useful treatments could be provided, leading to a change in the professionals' earlier expectations that certain patients were beyond saving. With higher expectations came the recognition that such patients needed more knowledgeable nurses and physicians. In America's post–World War II community hospitals, people died of hypovolemic shock, airway obstruction and respiratory failure, wound hemorrhage, toxicity from infection, starvation and dehydration due to obstruction (often the result of cancer), and a host of other immediate causes. Of these causes of hospital deaths, the ones most readily discovered and addressed by the expert yet simple vigilance of nurses seemed to be shock, airway obstruction, and wound hemorrhage.

By the 1950s, partly because of the availability of penicillin and its derivatives, cardiovascular diseases such as myocardial infarction (heart attack) and heart failure due to the effects of atherosclerosis had long since displaced infectious diseases as the leading causes of death and morbidity in the United States. Hospitals admitted large numbers of patients suffering from acute episodes of chronic diseases such as heart and vascular disease. At the time, estimates of the short-term mortality from acute myocardial infarction ranged from 30 percent to 40 percent; nearly half these deaths were caused by fatal irregularities of heart action called arrhythmias.[9]

In addition to those with medical illnesses, patients undergoing chest surgery, the then-novel heart-valve commissurotomy and replacement procedures, and vascular and large-scale abdominal surgeries experienced postoperative complications ranging from respiratory failure and shock to wound infections or wound drainage problems. These gravely ill persons overwhelmed the postoperative recovery room or private nursing care systems then in place. Ultimately, these surgical and cardiac patients, later joined by patients whose lives were prolonged by kidney dialysis, began to constitute a larger subpopulation of hospital patients whose demanding and time-consuming care requirements created a growing hospital nursing crisis.

At the same time, these gravely ill patients were coming to be evaluated by the public as "savable." Improved management and survival rates of seriously injured casualties during World War II and the Korean conflict of the early 1950s led to a new American optimism about emergency and intensive care for civilians. Patients and their families, as well as their doctors and nurses, thus began to share a different and much more expansive idea of routine treatment in the face of life-threatening, devastating illness. Expectations for successful treatment and care changed, but acknowledgment of the economic and social implications of meeting these new expectations happened only slowly. Hospital, professional, and community responses were framed and constrained by the unanticipated, unwanted expense of expanding nursing to achieve the kind of successful care people began to think possible.

The Nursing Care Dilemma

This increasingly complex patient population occupied overburdened hospitals in the midst of transition. Starting in the 1940s, hospitals slowly began to move away from a care system based on student labor and family-financed care given by private-duty nurses. The new graduate general-duty or staff nurses began to be paid, rather reluctantly, by the hospitals themselves. Hospitals enlarged their systems of staff nursing, partly in response to their public popularity and the rising public expectations of cure. But the way hospitals implemented new nursing models put critically ill patients at risk.

Forced to pay more for nursing services previously available at low cost, both hospital administrators and nursing leaders relied on management models premised on old assumptions. These models were based on the needs of the prewar, stable hospital population, which had included many convalescents and people recovering from relatively simple surgery such as appendectomy and tonsillectomy. Hospital supervisors and administrators assumed that nurses' work conditions and knowledge requirements would remain stable, and they thought that the growing number of nursing tasks could be offset by hiring more assistive workers. To control costs, hospital administrators hired less skilled person-

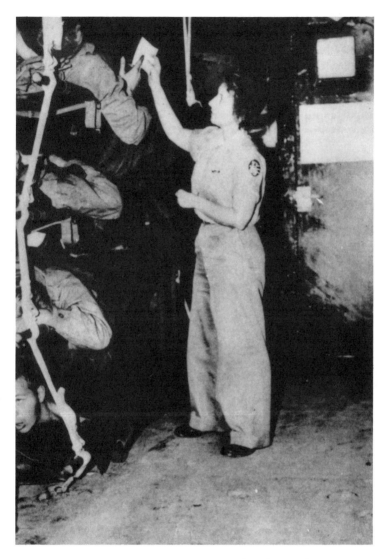

Figure 1. Nurse caring for Korean War casualties in transit to treatment in Japan. Courtesy of Joan Lynaugh, private collection, Bryn Mawr, Pa.

nel to extend the "hands and feet" of professional nurses, and they also searched frantically for ways to determine the lowest possible number of nurses needed to care for a standardized number of patients.[10]

Neither the problem nor the solution was merely a matter of numbers, however. The "hands and feet" solution failed because the assumptions on which it was based were wrong. The nature of the work of nursing, not simply the amount of tasks, was changing. Increasing patient complexity required a more flexible patient care workforce featuring greater numbers of nurses with many skills, rather than caregivers with the same or fewer skills. High rates of turnover and migratory work patterns of nurses, resulting in less experienced staff and diluted skill pools, complicated the caregiving situation.

Furthermore, the professional nurses who stayed on the job were insufficiently prepared to care for a more complex patient population. In the 1950s, 80 percent of nurses graduated from hospital-based educational programs that offered diplomas and qualified graduates to sit for state nurse-licensing examinations. Hospital-based training often was functional and task oriented. Education in physiology, pathophysiology, and pharmacology was usually rudimentary; nurses were expected to rely somehow on physicians' knowledge rather than their own to solve complex clinical problems. Nursing expertise usually developed on the job, especially in rapidly changing areas of practice such as cardiac and postoperative nursing.

Nurses were not the only caregivers lacking expertise to care for complex patients. Few of the nurses' physician colleagues were trained in the new trends in cardiology, and fewer still were familiar with rapidly changing advances in respiratory support. This is not so surprising; closed-chest massage to restart stopped hearts was introduced in 1959, closed-chest massage in tandem with mouth-to-mouth resuscitation in 1960, and direct-current defibrillation in 1962. Early coronary care units at Toronto, Kansas City, and Philadelphia were not established until 1962. Nonspecialist physicians who had received their training earlier were usually unfamiliar and uncomfortable with these innovations.

The Problems on the General Units

Nurses' work on the general patient care units was difficult and demanding. During the 1940s and 1950s, patient admissions to a unit were usually based on the nature of their diagnosis or the identity of their admitting physician. As a result, most patient care units housed a mix of patients, some capable of self-care or needing intermediate care and others needing postoperative observation or constant observation and care. When a patient was critically ill, the family might be encouraged by the nursing and medical staff to hire a private-duty nurse if they could find and afford one.[11] Often, however, families requested more private-duty nurses than could be found by the hospital.

Most of the time the nursing staff "made do." During the day, patient care was given by teams of nurses. The work was divided into specific tasks by the team leader, who was usually a registered nurse; a student or graduate nurse gave medications, and various nursing assistants and licensed practical nurses (LPNs) provided the rest of patient care. On a single unit there might be forty-five to sixty patients grouped into two or three clusters of fifteen to twenty per team. Each group might be tended by one or two graduate nurses, three or four students, and one or two LPNs or nursing assistants.

As has been noted, the patient care situation in the hospital of the 1950s and 1960s was very dynamic. On any single unit, patient conditions varied widely and changed rapidly. Often, inexperienced nurses faced new emergency situations with little assistance or appropriate knowledge. As one physician lamented, "Many nurses in their training and immediately afterward have been in contact with so few cases requiring intensive therapy . . . that they know relatively little about their management."[12] The combination of rapidly changing conditions and lack of preparation put critically ill patients at risk except during an immediate crisis—if it was detected.[13]

As Vickie Wilson reported in her 1990 retrospective on critical care, nurses in these situations felt they could not keep pace with their sickest patients or provide individualized care. One nurse recalled those years:

I remember having a patient on an Aramine drip. He was just across from the nurses' station, supposedly so I could keep a close eye on him. But

I also had 15 or 20 other patients with varying degrees of illness on my floor. I would run in to take a blood pressure; if it was all right, I would breathe a sigh of relief and go on to my other patients. When the drip needed titrating, I would speed it up or slow it down a bit [with a roller clamp] and hope for the best.[14]

These nurses felt guilty when their patients got into trouble, and when they faced such hectic conditions repeatedly they grew frustrated as well. All over the country, in erratically staffed but expanding hospitals, nurses found themselves responsible for desperately ill and dying patients whose medical and nursing needs exceeded the nurses' availability, knowledge, and authority. Left on their own to cope with these difficult and frustrating situations, some physicians and nurses were powerfully motivated to find a better way.

Early Models of Critical Care

Nurses, confronting daily crises caused by rising complexity of care needs among their patients, looked to the precedent of the postoperative "recovery room," introduced in the early 1920s but more common in the immediate pre–World War II period.[15] Usually located close to the operating suite, the recovery room provided transitional aftercare to patients undergoing major surgery. Each person was closely monitored while regaining consciousness after anesthesia.

The recovery room was a new approach to nurse staffing, representing one of the first times hospitals hired extra nurses for a particular group of patients because of specialized physiological need. It was an expensive effort for hospitals, but one more controllable than a hospital-wide initiative to improve staffing because the area was small and involved so few nurses. Before the development of the recovery room, postoperative or unstable patients remained on the wards and competed for attention from an overextended nursing staff.

The immediate predecessors of intensive care units were the polio units of the early 1950s, set up in response to the poliomyelitis epidemic in Europe and the United States. Treating paralyzed patients in the "iron lung" respirators required intensive supervision and care; gathering together patients with similar nursing care needs and assembling expert caregivers were logical and effective responses.[16] It would seem that the successes of these units might have been applied immediately to other categories of critically ill patients, but this did not happen. The emergency impetus of the epidemic disappeared, and hospitals hesitated to make the economic investment involved in long-term deployment of intensive nursing care and equipment.

During wartime, innovative medical and nursing care responses to the severely wounded developed out of necessity. In World War I, special units provided care to patients with particular widespread and severe medical problems such as gas toxicity and empyema. Special care for patients suffering from immediately life-threatening problems such as hypovolemic shock or thoracic wounds expanded during World War II. Rapid transport of injured soldiers and the availability of sulfa and penicillin for immediate treatment enabled medical teams to triage patients according to their ability to remain stable and benefit from more extensive treatment. Unstable casualties received more intensive care in field hospitals close to the battle. Each field hospital included a higher proportion of surgeons and nurses than did the evacuation hospital.[17] These developments were further refined during the Korean War, with the added advantage of even quicker casualty transport by helicopter.

Despite all this experience, the idea of creating a permanent special area for the care of critically ill patients was not institutionalized in civilian hospitals until intensive care units emerged in 1953. Although recovery rooms, polio wards, and field hospitals influenced the development of intensive care units, the concept was transformed into action only when the hospital environment and societal expectations of civilian medical care made it appear both practical and necessary.

Intensive Care Units

When we asked the nurses who founded the earliest intensive care units what they were attempting to accomplish, their responses were simple and straightforward. One said, "The units were invented because of the problems that came from a patient being desperately ill and needing *one* nurse. . . . Finding a way to respond to that situation multiplied by thousands of times forced us to change the hospital."[18]

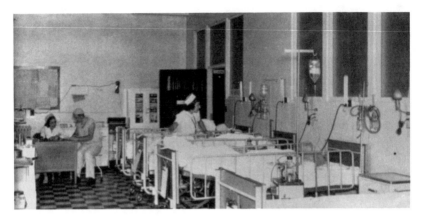

Figure 2. Intensive Care Unit, Veterans Administration Hospital, Hines, Illinois. Used with permission from *Modern Healthcare* (copyright Crain Communications, Inc.).

Faced with conflicting priorities for their services, dangerous care conditions, and a continuously rising demand for more hospital care, nurses and physicians turned to the familiar, traditional system of intense observation and triage of the most seriously ill. Long used in war and disaster to sort those most needy of care, triage favored patients with some promise of recovery. Two very old ideas were combined and refined to form the new idea of intensive care.

Intensive care units appeared in diverse geographic locations within months of each other in late 1953 and early 1954. In 1953 and 1954, the University of North Carolina Hospital in Chapel Hill, North Carolina, Manchester Memorial Hospital in Manchester, Connecticut, Albany Hospital in Albany, New York, Veterans Administration Hospital in Hines, Illinois, and Chestnut Hill Hospital all opened within months of each other. Hospitals and physicians apparently kept these developments to themselves for a while, and papers detailing how intensive care units worked were not quick to appear in the literature. The first published account of an intensive care unit appeared in the September 1954 issue of *Hospitals,* under the index heading "Recovery Room."[19]

Despite the diversity of their locations and the apparent absence of communication among them, the units were similar in four ways. Each grouped critically ill patients together in a designated space. The units were small (four to six beds), open rooms or a cluster of two to three semiprivate rooms with a common observation area. Each implemented more concentrated nurse staffing patterns than those found on the general floors. All provided twenty-four-hour, seven-day-a-week service.[20]

Later, some intensive care units (ICUs) appeared as part of a new system of hospital nursing care known as progressive patient care (PPC), first proposed in 1951 by the United States Army as a mechanism for patient classification and staffing needs assessment. The U.S. Public Health Service took the concept further in the late 1950s to reorganize the assignment of hospital patients according to the severity of illness. PPC called for four levels of patient care based on nursing care needs: special care or intensive care (later called critical care), intermediate care, self-care, and continuation care. Although PPC as a total system failed to gain public and professional acceptance, the ICU part of the concept flourished.[21] As Faye Abdellah, former assistant surgeon general with the U.S. Public Health Service, noted, "They [physicians] bought it immediately."[22]

Although ICUs and recovery rooms were built upon similar principles, the intensive care unit emerged as a distinctly organized, innovative patient care area. ICUs admitted patients from outside the hospital and from other units in the hospital in addition to those from the operating rooms. Unlike the recovery room, which usually closed in the late afternoon or on weekends, the intensive care unit stayed open all the time.

Although considered "new" areas, the intensive care units of the 1950s looked like small traditional wards.[23] As one nurse described an early unit, "You [just] take a big room . . . put a glass partition down through the middle . . . four beds at one end were partitioned off."[24] The units sprouted in available space such as closets or unused croup steam rooms. Not surprisingly, they were usually crowded, makeshift areas.

Down the hall we had two rooms that had a connecting bath. . . . What we did was put a piece of plywood over the bathtub and make us some cabinets or some shelves in the bathroom and we put a station in there with all the drugs and the supplies and a place for the doctor and nurse to sit to chart. . . . That way you didn't have to come out into the corridor and you could observe patients in two rooms.[25]

Such jerry-built units were the norm in the first phase of intensive care unit development.

The patient population also distinguished the intensive care unit from the general floor; intensive care units, in general, did not imitate the social and class stratification found in the hospital at large. The postwar private insurance boom tended to separate spatially the insured middle class, who desired newly affordable semiprivate rooms, from the uninsured lower classes, who were admitted to the wards and relied on the charity of various volunteer, state, and federal agencies.

The federally sponsored postwar building boom under the Hospital Survey and Construction Act (Hill-Burton) of 1946 further stratified general hospital care according to the ability to pay by encouraging construction of private or semiprivate rooms. The Hill-Burton Act also allowed segregation by race through "equitable provision": a hospital's racial segregation policies did not disqualify it from receiving federal funds as long as other community facilities cared for the excluded population.[26]

Intensive care units neutralized patient stratification in several ways, albeit with strings attached. Almost all units mixed female and male patients in one area, while strict social mores prevented mixing men and women on the regular wards. Most units admitted all races and all economic classes. For the poor, however, "free" care carried certain unacknowledged obligations. The poor submitted to the ministrations of students, interns, and residents in teaching hospitals or underwent new procedures, such as heart surgery, before physicians attempted these innovations on private patients. At times, the poor may have bargained for care by bartering autopsy permission for new treatments.[27]

There were other exceptions to egalitarianism in intensive care units. For example, many ICUs excluded terminally ill patients; as one author noted, ICUs "extolled the salvage rather than the failure."[28] Also, very wealthy patients easily afforded twenty-four-hour private-duty nursing coverage and recovered in their private rooms rather than in the intensive care unit. A few units excluded charity patients.[29] For the most part, however, intensive care units de-gendered, de-classed, and de-raced the care of the critically ill within an "unegalitarian and inherently rigid" traditional patient care system.[30]

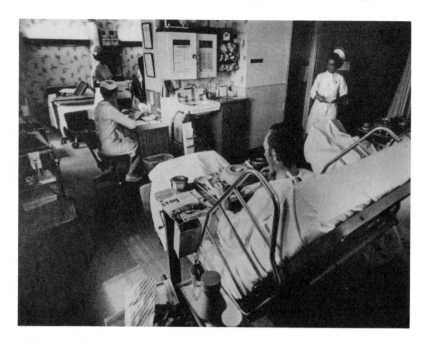

Figure 3. Concentrated nursing care, Anne Arundel General Hospital, Annapolis, Maryland, circa 1960. From *Planning for Cardiac Care: A Guide to the Planning and Design of Cardiac Care Facilities* (Chicago: Health Administration Press, 1973), 16. Used with permission.

Intensive Nursing Care

The characteristic of the new units that most closely resembled traditional attempts to safeguard physically unstable patients was the continuous presence of the nurse, who was constantly on watch: "You were sitting right next to the patients . . . they could hear everything. They felt safe because you were right there. I scared them to death when [I] went out of the room."[31]

In general, the units did not boast new or complex technology. The small space between beds, usually taken by oxygen tanks needed for tents, drainage bottles, and suction devices, indicated that planners did not anticipate the introduction of large, complex machinery. In fact, nurses who worked in the special care units

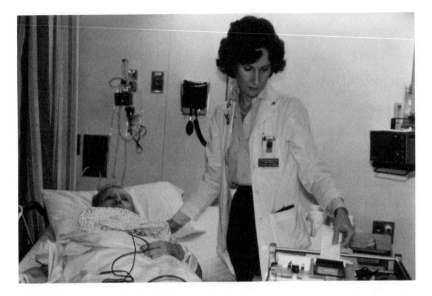

Figure 4. Specialized nursing care. Courtesy of the School of Nursing, University of Pennsylvania, Philadelphia, Pa.

of the 1950s recalled that they "didn't have any [technology]."[32] But they did; they used the same equipment as that used in the general units, such as blood-pressure devices, chest tubes, metal tracheotomy tubes, and catheters—"the old stuff"—but now it was gathered in one place.[33] Ethel Harrison, the nurse instrumental in developing the critical care unit at North Carolina Memorial Hospital, described her unit's success: "Though our beginnings were somewhat crude, the concept proved sound. . . . The parameters for monitoring patients then were principally the measurement of vital signs, the level of consciousness, intake and output, weight, the nurse's sense of hearing, sight, touch, smell, and sometimes her intuition."[34]

The nurses did not consider familiar equipment and machines "technology." To them, technology represented "new" science, machines (such as dialysis machines and heart monitors) that were complex and that actually kept patients alive or provided previously unobtainable data. These machines were incidental to the development of intensive care units. If early intensive care units contained monitors, they were not introduced into the hospital specifically for use in the intensive care unit. Technology came second; in fact, its full utilization was dependent on the reorganization of nursing practice.

The most obvious and distinctive feature of the intensive care units of the 1950s was the concentration of nursing care. The number of nurses working in ICUs of that era approximated the number assigned to a general hospital unit, but an ICU had a much smaller bed complement yielding a much higher nurse-to-patient ratio.[35] As Lawrence Meltzer, Rose Pinneo, and Roderick Kitchell noted in their 1965 guide to coronary care, "Intensive coronary care is primarily, and above all, a system of specialized nursing care [and its] success is predicated almost wholly on the ability of nurses to assume a new and different role."[36] The *Philadelphia Inquirer* told its readers in 1967, "Unless the nurse is capable of undertaking these extraordinary duties and responsibilities [identifying derangements in heart rhythms and understanding treatment for each disorder], intensive coronary care has limited value."[37]

Gathering the most ill patients together presented difficulties for nurses. The emotional context changed as the special units concentrated physically unstable, extremely ill patients in a small space. Nurses were confronted with an unrelenting stream of physiologically fragile, disfigured, often comatose patients and the daily occurrence of death.[38] The following is a composite from nurses who told us their critical care stories from the early years: "The patient is desperately ill . . . the physician couldn't come, didn't come, or didn't know what to do. The nurse swore . . . never again—I will learn what *they* know . . . about how the heart works, about defibrillation, about acid-base balance, about the interactions of drugs."

As they confronted the deaths of their patients, nurses urgently sought to learn more. Veteran critical care nurses frequently phrased their personal drive to learn in simple but urgent terms: "If you don't know what there is to know . . . you always think it is your fault [if something goes wrong]."[39] At first, nurses and physicians banded together for informal self-instruction sessions. Physicians taught the nurses physiology, pathophysiology, and how to read electrocardiographic rhythm strips and evaluate lab results. Nurses taught the physicians how the patients responded to treatment and what patient behavior to expect during the course of illness. As one nurse from Arkansas put it, "Doctors and nurses trained each other, and after a year or so the nurses were smarter than the doctors."[40] Nurses and physicians comforted each other when they made mistakes, and when, as often happened, they confronted failure, they wept together.

Mutual respect and collaboration between nurses and physicians in critical care involved adjustments and reconceptualizations on both sides. Cardiologists knew any improvements in patient outcomes rested on nurses' assuming broader clinical responsibility. Inevitably, that meant physicians would have to relinquish their traditional monopoly on clinical knowledge and decision-making. If patient survival was the goal, it was essential that nurses have the authority and expertise to diagnose and treat (by defibrillation) patients experiencing life-threatening arrhythmias. Thus, in a matter of months, nurses who previously had been forbidden to give aspirin for headaches found themselves restarting stopped hearts. Nurses reached an accommodation with physicians, a way to collaborate, by articulating a clear perception of critical care nursing, that is, intervening to stabilize the condition of unstable patients. Most important, nurses and physicians learned to trust each other as each practiced his or her own area of expertise.

The American Association of Critical-Care Nurses

By the late 1960s, small groups of intensive care nurses and coronary care nurses were meeting regularly, often in conjunction with their physician colleagues, to discuss clinical questions and intensive care unit management and to share professional concerns and problems with those knowledgeable about and sympathetic to their situations. These gatherings helped nurses obtain and verify needed information and skills they could not develop at their home institutions. Information—such as how to observe and interpret cardiac and respiratory problems, interpret electrocardiograms, investigate the rapidly developing monitoring technology, and become familiar with the new drugs coming into practice— was vital to their ability to care safely and effectively for their patients. In addition, the meetings gave nurses new confidence in their skills and in their influence on local and national trends. They found they were not alone, even though they were practicing outside the boundaries of traditional nursing.

In October of 1968, a large group of nurses met in Nashville, Tennessee, at a cardiac nursing symposium sponsored by physician colleagues and instigated by Norma Shephard, the director of the Cardiac Nursing Program at Baptist Hospital in Nashville. At the time, most of the nurses involved in critical care were still learning their skills on the job. Now, however, some began to offer continuing education courses to prepare other nurses for these demanding roles. The federal government and professional medical associations also sponsored training programs in coronary and intensive care nursing. A wide array of programs began to be offered, but there was little consensus about the knowledge nurses needed or their patient care decision-making responsibilities.

Shephard discussed the feasibility of an organization for nurses in intensive care with trusted nursing colleagues from five other states. She followed up on the 1968 meeting by sending roughly four hundred postcards to individual nurses inquiring about their interest in forming a national organization of cardiac nurses. Of the 131 nurses who responded, 127 supported the idea and 4 were opposed.

Many nurses wrote messages on their postcard responses: "Will be waiting eagerly to hear what I can do to help"; "I feel a great need for exchange of information with other cardiovascular nurses"; "I stand beside you 100%"; "Bravo! Send me 10 more cards." Encouraged by this response, Shephard called an organizational meeting in May 1969; the American Association of Cardiovascular Nurses was created in September of 1969.[41] The new organization attracted new members at an astonishing rate. In 1969, 140 nurses signed on; by 1970, there were 500 members. One year later, there were 2,800 members and twenty-six local chapters had been organized.

In 1971 the name of the organization was changed to the American Association of Critical-Care Nurses (AACN). The name change symbolized the struggle within the organization to include nurses working in all critical care situations, and not just those in cardiovascular nursing. It was the first in a series of foresighted moves toward inclusiveness that facilitated the AACN's remarkable growth in size and power. Today the AACN lists more than 75,000 members and draws as many as 8,000 attendees to its annual meeting, the National Teaching Institute (NTI). AACN is the largest nursing specialty group in the country.

The early leaders of AACN remember that they were hungry for camaraderie and knowledge. One remarked, "Our idea was that this was not just a passing fad, it is the future, nurses will [be the ones who] care for these folks."[42] Organization leaders sought out the American Nurses Association (ANA), investigating the option of becoming an interest group within the larger professional organization. The discussions were unsuccessful; the intensive care nurses wanted and needed to pursue a specialized educational and role-development agenda. They knew they had to respond to the rapid, unplanned, and rather dangerous escalation in clinical responsibilities placed on hospital nurses in the late 1950s or allow their practice boundaries to be determined by hospital administrators and physicians.

These changes in nurses' responsibility were already happening at the local, grassroots level. Changes in local practice preceded national debate. Yet to be decided were new standards of nursing education and nursing practice and the respective clinical responsibilities of physicians and nurses. The critical care leaders decided they had to define the new nursing role themselves.

An Expanding and Changing Institution

Intensifying care for critically ill patients took place within a context of an affluent Cold War society enthusiastic about modernizing and enlarging the United States health care system. Hospitals became one focus of this energy; optimism about better national health through applied, curative science paved the way for hospital expansion after World War II. The Hospital Survey and Construction Act (Hill-Burton) of 1946 provided capital for hospital development. Furthermore, the willingness and capability of hospitals to support intensive care units and the staff to care for an ever-expanding population of patients were newly grounded in a rich and growing private and public insurance system and the ideology of entitlement. Medicare and Medicaid became law in 1965; voluntary insurance systems like Blue Cross and Blue Shield continued to expand. The Regional Medical Programs of the Johnson administration's Great Society and hospitals' ability to pass educational expenses through to insurers helped defray the costs of additional education for personnel and expanding programs of care. In this optimistic, affluent, and expansionist period, it is no wonder that, by 1965, the intensive care unit idea had spread to more than a thousand of the nation's hospitals. By 1969, more than half the nation's not-for-profit hospitals claimed to have an intensive care unit.[43]

The post–World War II wave of institutional expansion and renovation created an architectural impetus for intensive care units. By the early 1950s, community hospitals generally abandoned their larger wards and built semiprivate or private accommodations for all of their patients. Even teaching hospitals, which traditionally had maintained large wards of indigent patients for teaching purposes, began to renovate their accommodations. Hospital planners hoped these changes would help them compete for paying patients by offering amenities such as privacy and quiet, previously reserved for wealthy patients. But housing critically ill patients in enclosed private rooms out of sight of the nurses created unanticipated risks. Newly renovated hospitals quickly had to rearrange their space again to facilitate gathering the sickest of their patients under the watchful care of expert nurses.

What was needed was a consensus about who should receive intensive high-cost medical and nursing care and who should not. What values would influence care decisions? Who was responsible for giving and overseeing care of the critically ill?[44] This book provides a lens through which the roots of our current idea of critical care nursing may be examined and suggests themes to inform contemporary debate and decisions. The history of critical care nursing in the United States reveals the multifactorial scientific, political, economic, and cultural forces influencing the development, definition, and provision of care to very sick people.

Chapter 2
Hospitals in Transition

Post–World War II United States hospitals underwent demographic, financial, architectural, and ideological changes that are still influencing contemporary health care policy decisions. Sicker patients entered hospitals for treatment and expected some sort of successful treatment, if not cure. Greater numbers of patients held some form of voluntary insurance and could afford hospital treatment. Hospitals, once solely dependent on charitable individuals for income and guidance, began to rely on individual clients and insurers for revenue and on professional administrators and the medical profession for guidance.[1] These changes provided the underpinnings for a major ideological shift in the public's perception of hospital care. The American public expected the hospital and its professional staff to do something for previously untreatable chronic illnesses and for this treatment to take place in a homelike setting rather than in warehouselike wards. To this end, the hospital became more than a place in which to recover from illness. It became a commodity in a competitive environment and began a metamorphosis to its contemporary form as a temple of expensive accommodations and life-saving treatments at the expense of preventive care.

Rising costs of hospital care in the 1950s, combined with falling endowments and paltry state aid, prompted loud discussions about the feasibility of continuing charitable or ward care on a large scale, especially in urban teaching hospitals. Although hospitals had steadily reduced their charitable orientation after World War I, philanthropic trustees and physicians in the 1950s found the shift from the charitable to the business mentality unsettling.[2] The shift proved even more troublesome for hospitals with physi-

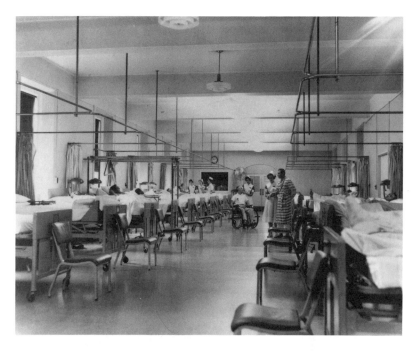

Figure 5. Ward scene, Philadelphia General Hospital, circa 1950. Courtesy of the Center for the Study of the History of Nursing, School of Nursing, University of Pennsylvania, Philadelphia, Pa.

cian training programs because it required a rethinking of the parameters of physicians' clinical training. Out of this conflict arose a hospital hybrid, a declassing of hospital accommodations and services, as all patients, no matter what their ability to pay, were placed in semiprivate or private rooms and interns and residents gained access to all patients during their training.

Although accommodations gradually became more egalitarian, covert stratification of patients by socioeconomic class remained. In 1968 Raymond Duff and August Hollingshead described the private accommodations as "away from the noise and clutter . . . windows provide a view of the residential sections of the city. . . . The rooms contain a built-in clothes closet, private toilet, washbasin. . . . The room is bright and tastefully decorated; it is furnished with a single bed. . . . The general impression is one of

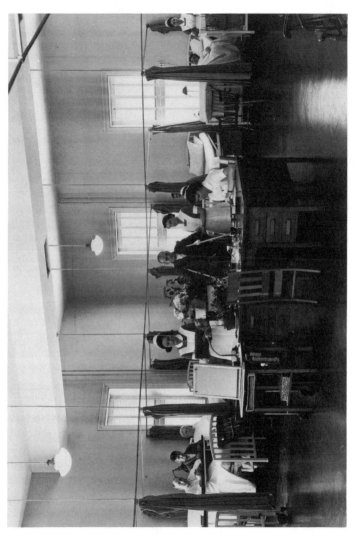

Figure 6. Ward scene, Massachusetts General Hospital, circa 1950. Most of the caregivers are students. Courtesy of Joan Lynaugh, private collection, Bryn Mawr, Pa.

light, airiness, and quiet."[3] In contrast, the remaining traditional ward accommodations are "in a building that has been characterized by the hospital authorities as obsolete. The halls are narrow and the rooms are dark. There are no private toilets or bathrooms or clothes closets. . . . The rooms are filled with beds which show the years of hard usage they have received."[4]

Stratification of patients was also exemplified by the category of physician care a patient received. Traditionally, the designation of "ward" acknowledged the patient's inability to pay or to buy privacy and symbolized the lack of choice. "Choice" was a class prerogative akin to privacy, because the type of accommodation determined the type of medical supervision. Access to private or semiprivate rooms indicated that the patient had the resources to pay and therefore could choose a private physician. Ward patients could not afford to pay and therefore could not choose their physician; ward patients received care from the "staff," an amorphous term that usually meant noncontinuous care from rotating groups of residents supervised by a cadre of staff physicians. Essentially, the terms ward (and later, service, when wards disappeared), semiprivate, and private described different patterns of care given to different classes of people. This meant not necessarily unequal medical care, but different patterns of continuity and access to physicians at different points in their careers.[5] One physician tacitly acknowledged the traditional stratification of care when he noted that, on Ward D, a patient's care "was such as would be received by very few private patients, even persons with unlimited means."[6]

Attempts to balance all needs (patient privacy, medical education, indigent care, financial solvency) fostered an emphasis on the privacy ideal as hospitals actively competed for middle-class, insured patients. Although it seems incongruous to suggest that free-care needs prompted and supported the growth of private rooms, the relationship is quite strong and longstanding. Government agencies allowed voluntary hospitals to expand their facilities, technology, and services through tax exemptions granted to nonprofit and charitable institutions (such as hospitals) and cross-subsidization.[7] Hospitals charged paying patients rates above the actual cost in order to subsidize ward care. Of necessity, hospitals entered the competition for paying, insured patients by offering

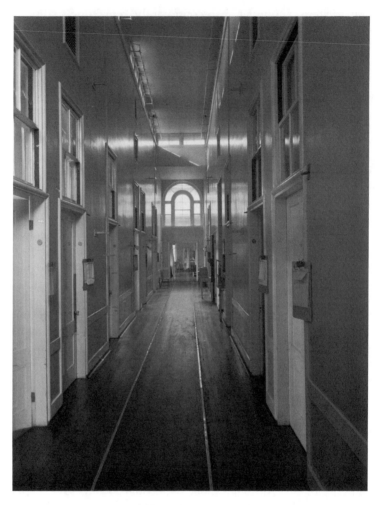

Figure 7. Philadelphia General Hospital private room corridor, date unknown. Courtesy of Joan Lynaugh, private collection, Bryn Mawr, Pa.

more attractive accommodations, better food, and, above all else, privacy traditionally reserved for the wealthy.

As hospitals moved to more intimate and enclosed semiprivate rooms, a conflict emerged between the hospitals' attempts to attract paying patients and the needs of an increasingly complex, critically ill patient population in hospitals. The change from predominately open patient care areas to the smaller, closed-off, semiprivate, and in many places all-private, rooms put the critically ill patient at risk because nurses could no longer easily provide a key element of care that these patients required—intensive and continuous observation.

Hospital planners and designers devised many strategies to improve nurses' view of the patient without compromising patient privacy. Most of these efforts focused on economizing nurses' time by shortening the distance of the hospital corridor or centralizing necessary supplies. Although these strategies proved helpful to nurses by reorganizing some of the functional aspects of nurses' work, they did little for the critically ill patient whose heart stopped or who began to hemorrhage out of sight of a busy nurse.

Although these changes occurred simultaneously at community institutions and academic centers, the way each institution responded to the changes reflected the ideology of each institution and the strength of the parochial forces initiating the change.

Increased Hospitalization

The hospital, especially after World War II, emerged as a strong symbol of growth reflecting American expertise and progress. The ability to "do something" for previously catastrophic illnesses solidified the hospital's position as the place in which to receive care and recover from illness. An impressive example of this effectiveness can be found in pneumonia and influenza death rates, which dropped from 108.2 deaths per 100,000 population in 1930 to 30 per 100,000 population in 1950, after penicillin became available to civilian hospitals on a large scale.[8]

The U.S. public's perception of hospital care evolved into a perception of health care as a "right" achieved through purchased or employer-provided private hospital insurance. In 1946, 30.3 percent of the civilian population had some form of private hospital insurance. This percentage rose to 44.6 percent by 1950, and to

74.1 percent by 1960.[9] The private insurance boom was supported in part by legal decisions such as the Inland Steel case of 1948, which allowed fringe benefits to be considered part of negotiable contracts, like wages.[10] Decisions in such cases provided hospital access for groups of middle-class people who previously had used hospitals only for emergencies.

Hospital utilization thus increased for various reasons: the rising number of insured persons, prevailing public beliefs in the ability of the medical professionals in hospitals to "do something," and the allure of technology and science, especially in the form of surgery, new procedures such as blood transfusions, and new medications. Between 1950 and 1960, admissions to short-term nonfederal hospitals rose 38 percent. A 7 percent decrease in the average length of stay, from 8.1 to 7.6 days, contributed to this trend, as did a 27 percent increase in the number of hospital beds. Occupancy rates during this period remained relatively stable: 73.7 percent in 1950, compared to 74.7 percent in 1960.[11]

Complexity of Care

In clinical terms, the majority of the hospital population was fairly stable during the 1950s. The number of admissions for acute illnesses such as pneumonia and influenza was almost halved by the end of the 1950s. Obstetrical deliveries and tonsillectomies were the first and second most frequent reasons for admission to hospitals during the same decade, but their combined percentage gradually decreased from 23 percent in 1946 to 18 percent in 1961.[12] Although the decrease does not seem dramatic, it was quite noticeable to caregivers in hospitals.

The number of sick and physiologically unstable patients in hospitals slowly climbed. The change was a function of two factors: a change in demographics and a change in the treatment offered to particular demographic groups. The hospital population was aging, supported in part by a growing proportion of aged persons who held some type of health insurance. This proportion increased from 26 percent of the over-sixty-five population in 1952 to 55 percent in 1963.[13]

Admissions of patients with chronic, debilitating illnesses associated with aging and the number of major surgical interventions for chronic illness increased. One study indicated that, from 1946 to 1961, the frequency of admission for acute coronary artery occlusion increased 155 percent; for diseases of the nervous system (e.g., strokes), 33 percent; for diseases of the digestive system, 8 percent; and for diseases of the bones and organs of movement (e.g., arthritis), 50 percent. Additionally, more of these patients were discharged alive.[14]

To more closely illustrate the changes occurring in hospitals, the records of two Philadelphia hospitals, Hospital of the University of Pennsylvania (HUP) and Chestnut Hill Hospital (CHH); were examined. CHH opened its intensive care unit in 1954, becoming the first ICU in the city and the state. Shortly thereafter, in 1955, HUP opened its unit. Both hospitals are voluntary, acute care, nonfederal hospitals, characteristics describing the largest group of general hospitals after 1945. In 1951, CHH, with 104 beds, resembled 32 percent of short-term, nonprofit general hospitals, but was close enough in size to be representative of the largest group of hospitals (less than 100 beds); HUP, with 685 beds, resembled 12 percent of hospitals.[15] Records from a twenty-five-year period, 1946 to 1970, were examined at both hospitals.

Surgeons at HUP performed an increasing number of major surgical procedures dealing with chronic, age-associated diseases such as heart and peripheral vascular disease, which indicated an older hospital population as well as wider application of these therapies. Although the number of surgical cases remained stable over a ten-year span (1950–1960), the case mix changed from a majority of minor cases (appendectomies, routine resections, tonsillectomies) to an even distribution of major (vascular bypass procedures, large-scale cancer resections, coronary valve and bypass procedures) and minor cases.[16] On the other hand, at CHH the number of minor cases remained stable (approximately 65 percent of the total cases), reflecting its position as a community institution rather than a university-based research or referral hospital. The total number of surgical cases in general, however, increased by 89 percent from 1950 to 1960.[17]

Public expectations of the possibility of receiving treatment for and surviving various physical problems changed. New medical and surgical procedures such as heart valve replacements and, later, coronary bypass procedures and dialysis were introduced for patients previously given little hope of treatment or survival. All groups involved in the hospitals—nurses, physicians, administrators, and the public—began to hold different perspectives on what constituted routine treatment for severely ill patients.

New medications and diagnostic procedures, and greater use of old ones, accompanied the changing pattern of care and patient population. One study reported, for the period 1946 to 1961, a 55 percent increase in the use of anticoagulants for coronary occlusions, the use of new, more potent medications such as Levophed and Aramine to maintain blood pressure, and a 30 percent increase in the use of electrocardiograms.[18] Patients undergoing surgical procedures were initially sicker, required "intensive" observation for shock, hemorrhage, and electrolyte disturbances, and were attached to more equipment such as chest tubes, intravenous lines, and tracheostomies. Another study noted that, from 1938 to 1953, there was a 900 percent increase in patients undergoing oxygen therapy, 177 percent more intravenous lines, and 56 percent more electrocardiograms.[19]

As more physically unstable and severely ill patients appeared in the hospital, nurses were confronted with more complicated and time-consuming procedures and conditions. Data from one "simple" task, morphine injections, exemplify the situation. The Pharmacy Committee at HUP determined that a simple morphine injection from a tablet took five to seven minutes to prepare (this did not include the time needed to find and identify the patient, inject the drug, clean the needles and syringes, or set up the hypodermic tray). The committee determined that nurses prepared injections using 15,500 tablets in 1956, requiring 1,291 hours of nursing time per year, or the equivalent of thirty-two eight-hour shifts, for this procedure alone.[20]

The care of patients undergoing oxygen-tent therapy represented another complex procedure requiring intensive nursing time and skill. Oxygen tents required twenty to thirty minutes of the nurse's time to assemble. Although technicians increasingly performed this work during the day, nurses were responsible for this task on the evening and night shifts at many hospitals. Oxygen-tent therapy required extensive monitoring of the patient's breathing, oxygen concentration, and humidity (the patient had to be kept dry) within the tent and of the functioning of the tent's mechanical parts (nurses had to make sure the motor and fan worked). Nurses performed most care through a small porthole in the tent; procedures had to be performed quickly and in groups of procedures to prevent oxygen loss.[21]

The penicillin-resistant staphylococcus epidemics and increased use of blood transfusions are two additional examples of the complex situations and time-consuming procedures facing nurses. Widespread civilian use of penicillin became possible after World War II, quickly reducing mortality rates from pneumonia and wound infections.[22] At HUP, preoperative use of penicillin skyrocketed to almost 70 to 80 percent of all general surgical cases in 1956, compared to less than 25 percent in 1950.[23] Penicillin-resistant staphylococcus infections began appearing at the hospital in the early 1950s. In 1951, the neurosurgery staff noted the devastating results of staphylococcus infection over the period of one month: one patient died and three children developed meningitis following lumbar puncture.[24] By 1957, the hospital reported twenty to forty cases of staphylococcus infection per month.[25] Several nurses and physicians suffered from large boils and lesions.[26] The infected patients required isolation from other patients to prevent spread of infection and reduce the incidence of secondary infection. For nurses, this involved the tedium of large-scale, time-consuming isolation routines, with the added danger of infection.

Changes in routine medical care also increased the complexity of care. Early ambulation (getting out of bed within no more than twenty-four hours after surgery) is one example. By 1952, more than 50 percent of surgical patients were ambulatory in two days, compared to less than 5 percent ten years before.[27] Most of these patients got out of bed at least twice a day, and most of them required assistance because they still were connected to drainage bottles and tubes. The following description provides a vivid picture: "[The patient] had two ureteral catheters that emptied into separate jars, one rectal tube with its receptacle, a Foley catheter that was connected to a drainage bottle, and a substantial perineal dressing."[28] Another nurse remarked, "It was not unusual for one patient to require a nurse to man the drainage bottles and tubes, along with one or two other people to support the patient. . . . You had to be a magician to do it."[29]

Early ambultion increased the possibility of mistakes and accidents. Medication administration took more time because nurses now had to find patients as well as ascertain their identification (hospital identification bracelets were uncommon until the late 1950s). The potential for patient falls increased, as those receiving pain medication wandered around hospital corridors not designed for patient traffic or encountered obstacles such as wet floors or equipment.

The increasing number of physiologically unstable patients also complicated nurses' work. A 1950 California study estimated that a ward of twenty-five patients contained several requiring the full attention of one nurse: an average of two patients returned to the unit after surgical procedures, 16 percent or four of the patients would probably be totally dependent (moribund, unconscious, paralyzed, or immediately postoperative), another four patients would be critically ill.[30] Estimates of the proportion of critically ill patients per general hospital ranged from 10 percent to 18 percent.[31] Just one critically ill patient took much of the nursing time allotted to a group of more stable or other critically ill patients.

In hospitals of the 1950s, nurses frequently faced new emergency situations with little assistance and experience as patient conditions rapidly changed. "Putting out brush fires" constituted the major focus of care as the amount and complexity of nurses' work overrode the boundaries of their preparation and their numbers. This meant that severely ill patients received intensive nursing care only during emergency situations, when something went wrong. The more stable patients were left to their own devices as nurses spent more of their time caring for the enlarging pool of critically ill. As Faye Abdellah, former assistant chief of the Division of Nursing Resources, U.S. Public Health Service, astutely noted, the "emergency became routine."[32]

Change in Ideology: The Philanthropic Mission and Postgraduate Education of Physicians

The traditional mission of voluntary hospitals included care for the poor or for those who did not have the resources to care for themselves; later, their mission expanded to the training of physicians. The philanthropic mission still informed hospitals of the 1950s but increasingly came under fire as hospital costs increased faster than did philanthropic funds and patient income. In 1946, national hospital revenues were only 4.4 percent higher than expenses for nongovernmental, nonprofit hospitals. By 1955, the margin had shrunk to 1.5 percent.[33]

Between 1930 and 1960, the proportion of hospital income generated from patient services increased. Nonprofit hospitals in 1955 received almost 91.4 percent of their total income from services provided to paying patients, including government and third-party reimbursement, compared to 83.5 percent in 1946.[34] At HUP, income from patient services climbed from 72 percent in 1942, to 83 percent in 1952 and 89 percent in 1959.[35]

The dollar value of income generated from philanthropic gifts remained relatively stable but declined in proportion to total income. Between 1935 and 1958, the proportion of income from philanthropy for short-term, nonfederal hospitals fell from 14 percent to 4 percent.[36] At HUP, endowments constituted 23 percent of hospital income in 1932, but fell to 8 percent in 1952 and 5 percent in 1959.[37]

As hospital expenses rose, the cost of ward care aroused frequent and active debate between boards of managers, who hoped for greater income, and physicians loyal to the hospital's benevolent mission and eager for the prestige of educating other physicians. At HUP, ward patients paid lower rates and fees than did semiprivate patients but used more services. Ward patients underwent an average of twenty-four laboratory tests per admission, compared to the semiprivate patient average of ten tests. Ward patients also underwent more radiologic examinations (six X rays per admission, compared to four) and remained in the hospital for longer periods of time.[38]

A number of factors contributed to the discrepancy in the use of services. Residents and interns supervised by staff physicians "learned" by practicing on ward patients. Additional and unnecessary tests may have been performed in an almost experimental manner for the sake of learning. Residents and interns rotated through the various wards on weekly or monthly schedules, depending on the service, offering patients little continuity in their medical care. Thus patients saw sequentially many different physicians, who ordered various tests according to their level of training and expertise. Additionally, ward patients may have been sicker, suffering from a greater variety of chronic diseases. Indigent patients could not afford preventive or maintenance care, and therefore came to the hospital only as a last resort during an acute illness.[39]

At HUP, ward patients averaged 45 percent of the total patient care days during the 1950s.[40] The large proportion of ward patients focused discussions about the construction of a new building at the heart of the ideological shift in hospital mission from benevolence and physician training to economic solvency. Because of the limited space available to the hospital, any new construction required demolition of old, large wards. Facing the loss of ward teaching beds, the medical staff protested, noting that the loss of ward beds would be "expensive" in terms of the "deleterious effect on the teaching of medical students and [would] lead to the failure to qualify for residencies in certain subspecialties."[41] Orville Bullitt, president of the hospital board of managers, addressed the concerns of these physicians at a medical board meeting: "It is the ward bed that is the expensive one. . . . I am becoming quite concerned about our financial operations."[42]

Although, by 1959, ward patients at HUP carried some type of hospitalization insurance or were eligible for public support, most of them left the hospital with an unpaid balance after treatment. The allowances granted by ward insurance or the state hardly approximated hospital-established ward costs.[43] For such reasons, hospitals passed on the costs of ward care to paying patients with private insurance through cross-subsidization, by increasing their room rates and fees for diagnostic tests and blood transfusions.[44]

Hospitals complained about the discrepancy between their established costs and payments from various agencies. For example, in 1951 the state of Pennsylvania allotted six dollars per patient per day for indigent care, which the president of the board of trustees of CHH noted "barely covered half of the actual costs for all [city] hospitals."[45] By 1964, voluntary hospitals in Philadelphia claimed they provided more than $7 million of care for indigent city patients but received only $1.6 million from the city.[46]

Because of the cost of ward care and the poor reimbursement received for it, the board of managers at HUP encouraged physicians to restrict admissions of indigent patients. The medical board, with a measure of agreement, noted:

The admission of medical indigent patients referred [to the hospital] must be evaluated before admission by their physician. If the patient presented particularly interesting teaching potential, the patient could be admitted to the clinic. If not, the patient is returned to his physician, with the information that for economic reasons, we are unable to undertake care for this patient.[47]

To the problem of cost of ward care at HUP was added the related problem of the shortage of semiprivate rooms. Through the early and mid-1950s, a growing number of physicians were situated, both geographically and financially, full-time at the hospital.[48] By 1956, more than 60 percent of physicians with admitting privileges practiced only at HUP.[49] Their incomes and their ability to devote time to charity cases depended on a reliable supply of semiprivate and private beds. Surgeons in particular complained about the lack of semiprivate rooms and noted that the number of surgical operations performed at the hospital between 1955 and 1961 remained relatively stable because the hospital could not accommodate their demands for semiprivate beds.[50]

Physicians at smaller community hospitals, such as CHH, also demanded more private and semiprivate beds for the same reasons as the university physicians. In a seeming contradiction, physicians at CHH also debated the addition of ward beds in the context of the need for an internship program.

Interns and residents were important to the hospital because most staff physicians had offices outside the hospital or traveled to several other hospitals during the day. Staff physicians, except for surgeons, spent little time in the hospital. Although physicians could be reached by phone, most were unavailable at night except in cases of emergency. Residents and interns staffed the hospital and emergency room in ways comparable to the service provided by nursing students. Just as nursing students were considered invaluable for the provision of nursing care, interns and residents were considered invaluable to the "proper [medical] staffing of the hospital."[51]

On the other hand, teaching residents and interns took time and was not rewarded at community hospitals. The director of the medical department at CHH spoke to these issues in his 1961 annual report:

The Medical Department members as a group . . . need to spend a surprisingly small percentage of their time in the hospital, and an even smaller percentage of their earnings is derived from hospital practice. . . . The medical doctor therefore who usually spends 70 or more hours weekly practicing away from the hospital contributes time [to professional activities] at the expense of recreational time with his family or by sacrificing income-producing office time.[52]

A surrounding community of middle-class rather than indigent people, the need for income derived from paying patients, and the relaxation of the quota of ward beds required by accreditation agencies for teaching purposes (provided that the staff make their semiprivate and private "case material" available to interns and residents) influenced CHH to increase the number of semiprivate and private rooms, rather than ward beds.[53]

The medical staff, trustees, and administrator of HUP came to similar conclusions. The hospital maintained its teaching program, of course, but slowly began to utilize all patients for physician education. One physician accurately acknowledged this trend:

[We] must face the fact that major trends in social betterment, which we can only applaud, are moving in the direction of a truly one-class society and the abolition of the class of individuals who are medically indigent. . . . We must study this problem to see how best medical education and training can be conducted in the absence of a medically indigent population.[54]

As the hospital decreased its proportion of ward beds, interns and residents slowly gained access to private and semiprivate patients for training. By 1960, the use of these patients for medical education purposes was generally accepted as the norm.[55] Concern about the number of ward beds declined, and a new wing that opened in 1962 contained only private and semiprivate beds.

The Privacy Ideal and the Competition for the Paying Patient

Privacy in hospitals has always been available to those who desired and could afford it and to some of those who needed it. Hospitals traditionally segregated from the general hospital population patients suffering from plagues, leprosy, or conditions found to be socially upsetting, such as disfigurement. Affluent patients depended on privacy to support their sense of well-being and comfort. Conversely, to those with medical conditions that required isolation, privacy could represent stigmatization.

Class perceptions and symbols traditionally pervaded hospital accommodations. As one administrator noted, "Only the poor liked wards."[56] Traditionally, private rooms in hospitals were always available for the wealthy; many nineteenth-century hospitals created finely appointed rooms to attract out-of-town wealthy visitors without family to care for them during their illness. Private rooms separate from the general ward areas allowed affluent clients to maintain their distance from the common people, as they did in their homes.

Relaxation of the social stratification of patients in hospitals occurred during times of economic hardship, such as the Depression of the 1930s when few could afford the luxury of private accommodations. During this time, the concept of the semiprivate room emerged as hospitals broke up unused private suites into smaller, plainly decorated, multibed rooms to be used by the growing middle-class population. By the 1940s and 1950s, the large wards of thirty to fifty patients had disappeared except in large urban hospitals. By adding partitions, the large wards became smaller wards of eight to twelve beds or semiprivate rooms of up to six beds.

Despite the breakdown of the wards, hospitals continued to stratify accommodations in various ways. For example, a combination of private rooms (usually clustered around a nursing station), semiprivate rooms, and intermediate wards (usually at the far end of the hall) might have constituted one type of unit. The same hospital, built vertically as a facsimile of a hotel, might have located an entire unit of private rooms on the top floor of the building, in a manner akin to a penthouse suite. Units of semiprivate rooms might have been located on the middle floors, and "free" or service beds on the lower floors.[57]

Hospital construction from the mid-1940s reflected trends found in suburban housing construction. For example, new suburban homes in the 1950s had more bathrooms to ensure the privacy of each family member. Designs included powder rooms for guests to minimize visitors' use of the owners' bathroom, baths attached to master suites, and separate spheres for recreation and "living" (e.g., living room, dining room). These innovations effectively created the seclusion and privacy preferred by the newly affluent suburban home buyer.[58]

Hospitals appropriated these designs to maximize the hospitals' appeal to paying patients. Patients could now expect comfort and privacy similar to that in their own homes. Hospitals constructed in the 1940s and 1950s tended to have a bathroom in each room. Rooms had fewer beds, usually two to four per room, with space for dining and conversing with visitors.

All-private-room hospitals also proved popular for both economic and social reasons. The secretary of Health, Education, and Welfare urged state Hill-Burton agencies to encourage the construction of private rooms to maintain higher occupancy figures. By doing so, a community required fewer beds.[59] Although the initial construction cost might be higher than that for a multibed-room hospital, private rooms held other benefits—for example, they offered greater privacy and flexibility, shielded patients from depressing scenes, eliminated roommate incompatibility, and allowed for less costly transfers. As one HUP committee noted, "Separation of indigent and nonindigent patients is automatically provided and the dignity of the patient is preserved regardless of economic status."[60]

The changes in accommodations also conveniently facilitated therapeutic innovations. More intimate rooms with convenient bathrooms helped nurses manage new therapeutic interventions, such as earlier ambulation after surgery. Closer bathrooms (large wards had bathrooms outside the immediate ward area) encouraged gradual mobility, from the bedside to the bathroom and eventually to the hall. Easily accessible bathrooms allowed patients to depend less on devices such as bedpans and bedside commodes and gave nurses easier access to cleaning facilities when patients used equipment.[61]

Again, as was the case for suburban housing construction, hospital planners attempted to achieve the most privacy at the least cost. They accomplished this by attempting to do more, to achieve a degree of privacy and include a greater number of beds, in less space. The placement of beds, correct width of doorways, and need for windows figured prominently in debates about semiprivate and private room accommodations. Studies in the fields of psychiatry, which indicated that patients preferred corner beds for security, and of space travel, which evaluated the amount of space needed to prevent a feeling of confinement, contributed to room designs.[62]

The growing pool of privately insured patients provided the strongest economic incentive for semiprivate room construction and, indirectly, the continued stratification of patients by socio-economic status. Private insurance companies such as Blue Cross or Nationwide, covering the largest group of insured patients, fully reimbursed patients or provided them a room allowance for stays in semiprivate rooms. By 1945, more than 70 percent of Blue Cross contracts provided these incentives.[63] Patients who had previously only had the option of ward accommodations now chose two- to four-bed rooms and paid physicians and incidental expenses from their personal savings.

Consumers showed a clear preference for semiprivate rooms, as seen through the popularity of semiprivate insurance contracts. Blue Cross began offering ward-accommodation contracts in 1939, but discontinued most of them by 1945 due to lack of consumer interest.[64] Physicians shared and reinforced the preference for private or semiprivate rooms for their patients. To the chagrin of hospital administrators, some physicians at HUP advised their private patients to stay out of the hospital when semiprivate accommodations were unavailable, to protect them from the "hazards of the wards."[65]

Because of their reliance on patient income, hospitals depended on the local community to use hospital facilities. Hospitals therefore struggled to capture the loyalty and attention of the community by creating an attractive image worthy of community support. This strategy involved "putting a spin" on science. Not only did hospitals attract patients in ways likely to support reimbursement and provide better medical care, such as employing renowned physicians and using advanced technology, but they did this within an environment of wonderful decor, large rooms, or hotel-quality food service.

If patients had to wait for admission to the hospital or if they were admitted to rooms considered substandard, they might find another physician or hospital in the city. Philadelphia suburban hospitals presented even greater competition as people moved out of the city during the 1950s. Suburban hospitals provided excellent medical care, usually by HUP-trained physicians, and new hospital facilities without the complications of urban health care.[66] One father, who happened to be a major contributor to HUP, wrote to his daughter's physician: "By the way, the room first given [my daughter] in the dilapidated old section of the hospital with no private bath was enough to put anyone in the dumps. . . . Naturally the question arises in my mind as to whether the [hospital] is so over-crowded that some other hospital might not be a better proposition for the future."[67] The physician, in turn, wrote to the chief of surgery: "It is really impossible to practice proper medicine here with the facilities of my only hospital so hard to obtain and so uncertain. . . . We often lose patients to other institutions and other doctors because of our inability to get them into the [hospital]."[68]

Architectural Changes and Nurses' Work

The shift to predominately semiprivate and private rooms occurred at the same time that hospitals experienced increased utilization and their patient population grew more complex. This three-way change presented grave consequences for the care of the critically ill patient and the organization of nurses' work. First, putting walls between patients and nurses, no matter how many beds per room, prevented easy and constant observation of patients by nurses and put patients at risk. John Thompson and Grace Goldin accurately noted in 1975 that privacy always meant a sacrifice of continuous supervision.[69] Second, nurses' work moved from the patient's room (the general ward) to the hallways between rooms. Nurses spent more of their precious time walking from room to room, in part because hallways were longer, supplies were less centralized, and they could no longer easily observe their patients or the workers and students they supervised.

Mary Clymer, in her student diary in December 1887, wrote of the difficulties of patients in private rooms:

Got dressings ready for three antiseptic cases, still taking care of four patients. Trying to have my eyes in thirteen while my hands make a bed in eleven. The patient in thirteen has to be watched, the one in eleven is so afraid of a draught that I have to keep the door closed.[70]

In 1974 William McClenahan, a Philadelphia physician, also described the hazards of more contemporary semiprivate rooms:

In recent years, for perplexing reasons, it has become the fashion to maroon sick people in private or semiprivate rooms. . . . What unconscious patient can ring a bell when he needs assistance? Who is to know of his need? What companion—other than an occasional visitor—is there to re-lieve loneliness and fear, the two common denominators of illness?[71]

Wards allowed nurses to observe patients easily from just about any point in the room. Nurses considered this ability extremely important because continuous observation of patients constituted a key component of patient protection. Unobstructed observation of patients prevented accidents. For example, continuous obser-vation enabled a nurse to see a restrained and demented patient attempting to climb over the bed rails. The nurse could offer assis-tance before the patient fell or was otherwise harmed.

The opportunity to maintain vigilance even when busy with other patients provided a sense of relief to nurses and safety to patients. Open wards of any size allowed nurses to observe the critically ill patient at any time without necessarily traveling to the bedside. Important signs such as skin color, condition of ban-dages, or agitation were generally easily observed and acted upon even by an extremely busy nurse. Without the opportunity of con-tinuous observation, nurses feared they could not protect their patients. One nurse reported her fears of being unable to see or hear her patients:

I can remember as [a] student working on the cardiology unit where you had a lot of patients who came in with heart attacks. We would make rounds at night in those rooms just hoping that they would be alive. . . . We had to go around with flashlights and go into their room. We would go up to the bedside and count their pulse . . . check their breathing.[72]

As hospitals deskilled their work force in the 1950s by hiring nonprofessional workers, professional nurses spent more of their time in supervision and instruction. Semiprivate and private rooms made supervision less effective because nurses could not easily see or find the workers. The same problem occurred with nursing students, who relied heavily on professional nurses for supervi-sion and demonstration. A report from the 1959 National League for Nursing's consultation visit to HUP's School of Nursing con-firmed the difficulties of student supervision on private and semi-private floors. The spatial setup of the private floors was "a prob-lem," the report noted, because students could not be observed. If the school utilized these units as clinical settings, the report continued, more instructors would be needed to ensure adequate supervision and instruction.[73]

The move to smaller rooms also eliminated the invaluable informal patient reporting system. On the wards, while nurses were busy with a critically ill patient, more stable patients reported the problems of their fellow patients, helped sicker patients with bedpans, or adjusted their bedcovers. One nurse suggested that patient reporting "was like having a second pair of eyes and ears" and was sorely missed on the semiprivate units.[74]

To overcome the difficulties of enclosed rooms along long hallways, nurses relied primarily on their traditional method of safeguarding critically ill patients—patient triage. If the central room of a patient unit happened to be a two- or four-bed room, one nurse provided care to a group of critically ill patients. In these situations, nurses pooled supplies and general equipment in one room for a group of patients.[75] Ironically, on semiprivate and private units the nursing station no longer held the strategic importance that it had on the ward. Because of the solid-walled hallways, nurses had to travel to the patients' rooms to assess their condition. Although grouping critically ill patients close to the nursing station decreased a nurse's travel time, it did not offer the same opportunity for intensive observation.[76]

Although all agreed on the need for nurses to see their patients, few devices and innovations addressed the problem helpfully. One exception was the use of glass partitions on the wall facing the hallway. The Falkirk Ward, in Edinburgh, Scotland, had glass partitions from the ceiling to the mattress level on the corridor wall of the rooms situated next to the nurses' station, which were usually used by physically unstable patients. Intermediate-care rooms, further down the hall, had glass to the shoulder level of the nurse. Rooms for stable patients had no glass.[77]

Most solutions did not directly provide greater ability to observe patients. Instead, the solutions focused on maximizing the efficiency of nurses while they performed the functional aspects of their work. As Thompson and Goldin noted, "Every step [of a nurse] became a precious commodity."[78] Hospital planners experimented with alphabet floor plans (e.g., H-, T-, O-, X-shaped floors) to decrease corridor lengths and travel time for nurses. Architects had the double duty of reproducing the number of beds found in wards in semiprivate or private rooms along a single or double corridor. Devices such as the Nurseserver, various call-bell systems, and in-wall oxygen and suction outlets appeared in hospital rooms, theoretically to improve the efficiency of the nurse but not necessarily the nurses' view of a group of patients.[79]

Mechanical systems proved poor substitutes for the personal observation and supervision of patients by the nurse. For example, for a call-bell system to work, a nurse had to be present at the central call board at the nurses' station. But on units of semiprivate and private rooms, nurses no longer gathered in that location. Nurses were in patients' rooms or in the hallways.

By the 1950s, acute care hospitals in the United States consisted primarily of semiprivate and private rooms designed to accommodate stable patients such as those undergoing herniorrhaphies or tonsillectomies. Within a stable health care environment, changes in hospital accommodations should not have made a great difference in the way health care was provided. However, hospitals of the 1950s were in flux. Increased hospital utilization, primarily by a growing population of insured patients, and an increasingly complex patient population provided an unstable base for architectural changes.

These changes occurred in response to the community's desire and ability to pay for smaller, more private accommodations and hospitals' attempts to fulfill the community's needs. Neither group, however, had bargained for the risks entailed in the move to predominately semiprivate and private rooms. Putting up walls prevented nurses from observing their patients and therefore prevented quick responses to critical incidents. Patients hemorrhaged or fell out of bed, out of sight.

Chapter 3
Nursing in Transition

Eleanor Lambertsen, a post–World War II nursing leader, noted that "in 1938 [we were] still studying whether we needed graduate nurses in hospitals. . . . After the war there was no question . . . but also no nurses."[1] Although there was a national consensus after the late 1940s that nurses were central to hospitals' responsibility to provide care to patients, there was little agreement or understanding about the exact nature of nursing care or the knowledge needed to provide it.

Hospital staff nursing in the decade 1950 to 1960 was a "young" occupation still functioning according to traditionally defined visions of nursing care despite changes occurring in hospitals.[2] Nurse training schools adequately prepared nurses to care for most patients in hospitals—physically stable patients undergoing diagnostic studies, tonsillectomies, or hernia repairs—but not for physically unstable patients.[3] Staff nurses working in hospitals survived by gaining expertise through episodic exposure to various patient conditions or by trial and error. The idiosyncratic experiences of these nurses essentially determined how most nurses were trained and what they should know, because those who survived went on to be the head nurses, supervisors, and instructors responsible for the educational experiences of students.

Various studies of the nursing profession provide a context for the struggle to answer the question, "What is good nursing care?" The best known of these, Esther Lucile Brown's *Nursing for the Future: A Report for the National Nursing Council* (1948), and numerous other studies of nursing functions, working conditions, and job satisfaction emerged during this time.[4] The reports shared several conclusions: first, the work of nurses in hospitals had grown beyond the level of the knowledge and skills of a limited staff; second, heterogenous levels of nursing care workers provided care to patients; and third, disorganization and ineffective utilization of nurses occurred in the absence of a clearly defined, consistent concept of nursing care in both nursing education and nursing practice. In a stable care environment, these factors might have been addressed systematically. Within the rapidly changing hospital environment, however, they became exaggerated and disruptive.

Schools of nursing were unable and, at times, unwilling to keep up with the fast pace of new knowledge dissemination in hospitals. Until the late 1940s, the nursing education system still prepared nurses primarily for personal care and case-oriented private-duty or visiting nurse positions. Most of the staff nurses working in hospitals in the 1950s were products of the atomistic, procedure-oriented, and diagnosis-centered type of education system found in hospital training schools. Nurses learned, through frequent repetition, how to carry out basic essential personal care such as patient bathing and procedures such as bandaging and medication administration. They learned about signs and symptoms of various diseases, anatomy, physiology, and morbidity figures, but not the meaning or relationship of these subjects to the patient's condition. Nurses were not expected to relate the various observations they made to the patient's condition. One nurse noted, "We knew how to measure but not if we were measuring the right thing. . . . We knew he was alert and we knew he was in pain."[5]

Nurses' Skills and Knowledge

Several studies demonstrated the limits of nurses' knowledge. A 1951 study of Washington state nurses indicated that some nurses lacked the knowledge to take patient histories or counsel patients, and some were not trained to work with intravenous fluids, blood transfusions, or different suction devices. Although some of the procedures, such as administering intravenous medications and monitoring blood transfusions, were skills newly assigned to nurses, the study indicated that more recent graduates as well as older graduates were untrained in these areas.[6]

A later study (1967) by Elmina Price indicated areas of deficiency in skills and knowledge of nurses in both direct care (56.6 percent of nurses surveyed reported problems related to the care of a specific patient) and indirect care (33.6 percent reported difficulties in management-leadership skills and 43.7 percent reported problems dealing with interpersonal relations). In self-reports of critical incidents related to direct care, nurses pointed to a lack of knowledge and skills in the care of patients undergoing cardiac arrest, patients in labor in the delivery room, patients recovering from heart surgery, and patients exhibiting behavioral problems.[7]

Nurses coped with their knowledge limits by establishing time-consuming routines to assure themselves of their patients' safety. Awakening patients at 6 A.M. for temperature, pulse, and respiration measurement (TPR) is one example of a routine that provided a harried night nurse with a psychological "cushion"; seeing the patient at 6 A.M. and documenting the visit through TPR relieved the nurse of responsibility if something went wrong on the day shift.

Routines involving these three measurements became the hallmark of patient safety to nurses who did not fully understand the relationship between their observations and their patients' conditions. Based on previous observations, the nurse should have been able to decide if patients needed a 6 A.M. assessment or uninterrupted sleep. Instead, nurses without the expertise or authority to make these decisions relied on time-consuming and meaningless routines that had more psychological than medicinal value.[8]

The limits of nurses' skills undermined the quality of care that patients received. Unable to understand the relationship of certain signs and symptoms, nurses could not easily anticipate changes in a patient's condition or plan the next stage of response. For example, a patient receiving a blood transfusion required observation for chills, change in temperature, and headache. Although nurses easily observed and documented these symptoms, they had to learn through experience that the symptoms signaled a transfusion reaction and know what to do about it.[9]

Because of the undefined and inconsistent parameters of nurses' work, staff nurses required supervisors and head nurses with the appropriate preparation and skills to help them adapt to hospital-based practice. Most hospital head nurses and supervisors, however, advanced through the ranks on the merits of their clinical expertise rather than on their management skills. Most head nurses learned how to prepare and plan staffing schedules and supervise several groups of nursing care workers the same way they ac-

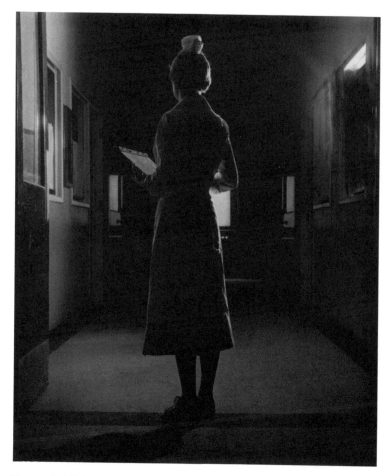

Figure 8. Night supervisor, Philadelphia General Hospital, circa 1950. Courtesy of the Center for the Study of the History of Nursing, School of Nursing, University of Pennsylvania, Philadelphia, Pa.

quired clinical expertise, through trial and error. Ironically, once in their management positions head nurses relinquished most of their clinical practice, thus denying less skilled nurses important role models.

Specialists (the term applied in the 1940s and 1950s to the ranks of educators, supervisors, and administrators) with adequate skills were difficult to find. Brown, in 1948, noted the "hundreds of positions carrying maximum salary and prestige in the supervisory, planning, administrative categories . . . either unfilled or filled by persons of inadequate ability or preparation."[10] A 1954 study of Michigan hospitals revealed that 71 percent of the supervisors of nursing care lacked general education past high school and nursing preparation past the diploma. Five percent had not completed high school.[11]

The Scope of Nurses' Work

Nurses needed skilled leaders not only to help them acquire clinical skills but also to help organize their growing workload. In 1958, Everett C. Hughes and associates described the scope of the roles professional nurses held in hospitals as teachers, administrators, and organizers.[12] In fact, professional nurses did just about everything, from mowing the lawn at one small Kansas hospital to setting up patients in respirators.[13] Nurses were trained and expected to move easily between various levels of responsibilities. Claire Dennison, in a spot study, described the number, variety, and complexity of procedures and treatments performed by nurses, as well as the various levels of responsibilities that nurses assumed. Over a twenty-four-hour period at a large teaching hospital with an average census of 473 patients (not including the operating room and labor and delivery rooms):

[One hundred nine] were ordered blood pressures in intervals of every fifteen minutes to once a day. Sixty patients, or one patient in every eight, received parenteral fluids or transfusions . . . and required constant attendance. . . .

They applied sterile compresses and painted lesions. They did approximately 230 dressings . . . and this does not include the times these dressings were taken down to show the wound to a surgeon. . . . They administered approximately 1,500 medications daily . . . by mouth or hypodermic. . . . They taught patients and their families to give insulin. . . . They had an average of seven patients a day under oxygen therapy. . . .

While all this went on, they met the usual expectations of the staffs. . . . It was understood that the nurses would know how to administer any drug—and pick up any error in writing the order.[14]

A 1950 study of California nurses indicated that, on a ward of twenty-five patients, nurses undertook an average of seventy-four new physician orders, administered forty-eight parenteral medications, made ten occupied (by patient) beds, and performed sixteen singular procedures (e.g., enemas, eye washes), among other things, over a twenty-four-hour period.[15]

Not all nurses' work related directly to patient care. As Dennison noted, "Nurses [are] considered an extension of all the services of the hospital."[16] It would have been "inconvenient" to all concerned if nurses had not known how to operate certain equipment or the workings of departments other than nursing (especially in the evening or at night when departments such as dietary service or pharmacy were closed). In 1954, the nursing supervisor also served as the night administrator at 66 percent of hospitals with 500 or more beds and 77 percent of hospitals with 100 to 199 beds.[17] Although this trend appeared to wane in the 1960s, a 1966 study indicated that, in 80 percent of hospitals surveyed, nursing supervisors still covered central supply or pharmacies. In 18 to 21 percent of hospitals, housekeeping and dietary service were administered by nursing supervisors during evenings and at night.[18] At Hospital of the University of Pennsylvania (HUP) in Philadelphia, nursing supervisors, not pharmacists, obtained medications for patients at night. The pharmacy committee noted that nursing supervisors made an average of ten trips a night to secure emergency drugs.[19]

State nursing associations commissioned nursing function studies during the 1950s that also documented the broad scope of nurses' work and the difficulty in defining that work.[20] Diverse results of the nursing function studies revealed the difficulties nursing leaders encountered while trying to establish a national consensus about "good" nursing care. Differing results due to geographic region and hospital size indicated that nursing care was defined on a local and contingent basis. However, several trends did emerge from the studies: nurses spent a lot of time performing physician-ordered physical care of patients (giving medications, changing dressings), keeping the nursing unit in order (stocking cabinets, counting supplies), and completing records (nurses' notes, requisition forms, reports). Nurses did not have a lot of time to intensively observe critically ill patients.[21]

The type of work nurses performed contrasted with the type of work nurses preferred. One study suggested that more than half of the nurses sampled desired more time for bedside nursing.[22] A Washington state study indicated that 54 percent of the sample found bedside nursing to be the most satisfying part of nursing.[23] Leonard Reissman and John Rohrer's 1957 study of a large southern university teaching hospital found that nurses preferred their work to have a mix of both technical tasks and bedside care; the four tasks preferred most highly were administration of oral medications, applying a bandage to a patient, making a patient's bed, and assisting a patient to walk.[24] Another study of three southern hospitals derived similar conclusions. In this particular study, both head and staff nurses highly ranked procedures such as administration of oral and intravenous medications and dressing changes. Staff nurses, however, ranked tasks that allowed personal contact with patients, such as bathing patients, keeping patient rooms tidy, and answering call lights, as highly as the preferred technical tasks.[25]

Work Organization and Staffing

The contrast between the work nurses performed and that which they preferred may be explained by the fast pace and high volume of their tasks and the method of work organization. The time nurses actually spent with patients was segmented into functional tasks; team assignment became institutionalized only in the mid-1950s, and then as a mix of functional and case assignment.[26]

When nurses organized their work by the functional method, tasks such as administering medications or treatments became the sole responsibility of a particular nurse. An additional nurse, if present, was usually assigned the care of a large group of patients, including those most physically unstable. Auxiliary workers or students may have assisted this nurse and provided a large portion of the routine personal care, such as feeding patients and bedmaking.

Nursing care took on an assembly-line character: a patient received a bath from one person, medications from another, and dressing changes from someone else. Patients interacted with professional nurses inconsistently, usually only during medication administration or treatments and with several different nurses on several different schedules. Beyond physical measures, nurses did not have much opportunity to offer patients other types of care—in particular, psychosocial care. Esther Lucile Brown pointed out the deficits of this system in which "a graduate or student nurse is detailed to give medicine to each patient for whom it has been prescribed the length of the ward, and other nurses are detailed to give treatments. Who is detailed to sit beside patients . . . and give a form of nursing care that may be more important than medicine or treatment?"[27]

Functional nursing helped understaffed nurses "get the work done," especially within a constantly changing and busy hospital work environment.[28] Available time, number of patients, and procedures, rather than the needs of the patient, became the regulators of tasks. One nurse recalled the staffing ratio at a southern hospital during the mid- to late 1950s as one nurse per twenty patients.[29] A 1953 nursing text suggested the use of two teams per forty patients; each team included a graduate or student nurse, a licensed practical nurse, and an orderly.[30]

One nurse described her evening experience on a medical ward in the early 1950s at HUP:

There was a whole ward full [thirty-two patients], two to four patients on a back porch, two beds outside in the hall opposite the utility rooms, and six more beds across the hall in a semiprivate area. And there were just the three of us to take care of them . . . myself and a senior student and maybe an orderly . . . who was a bit slow but a very nice older man. . . . I would find myself walking home up to Forty-sixth and Spruce at two or three in the morning. . . . We didn't get paid overtime or extra vacation time. That's the way it was, you just put in the overtime.[31]

During the mid-1950s at the same hospital (on the day shift), there may have been two professional nurses assigned to a ward of thirty patients: a head nurse and a general-duty nurse who administered all the medications and performed the more complicated treatments and procedures. One or two aides, an orderly, and several students usually assisted the professional nurses.[32] A 1958 staffing survey at the hospital revealed that, over a twenty-four-hour period in May on Ward D, one head nurse, one assistant head nurse, two graduates, one practical nurse, and two second- or third-year students provided care to forty patients. A private floor with forty-three beds had two head nurses, seven graduates, five practical nurses, and eight freshman students scheduled for duty over the same twenty-four-hour period, in addition to private-duty nurses. An average of 104 general-duty nurses, 56 practical nurses, 108 private-duty nurses, and 87 students provided care to

742 patients over twenty-four hours.[33] Although 104 nurses may seem adequate, this number is artificially high because it included 28 nurses assigned to the operating room and to the outpatient and emergency departments who were not available to shore up the unit staffing.

At Chestnut Hill Hospital (CHH), the nurse-patient staffing ratio appeared somewhat reasonable during the day but was overwhelming and dangerous on the night and evening shifts. Staffing levels changed according to the number of students available for clinical work. For example, in 1952, when only twenty-three junior and senior students remained in the school, night and evening professional nurse staffing was at its highest level. In 1954, eighty-two students were available for clinical work. As a result, evening and night professional staffing levels dropped and remained low until after 1956, when the school received only a temporary accreditation rating from the National League for Nursing (NLN). Professional staffing on these critical shifts improved during the next year despite a continued high number of students in the school.[34]

Low nurse-to-patient ratios proved potentially dangerous for critically ill patients. Patients with tetanus, bleeding esophageal varices, or congestive heart failure all could have ended up on one unit at the same time, and each of these patients required the constant attention of one professional nurse. One nurse described an incident that occurred while she attended another patient:

This man with bleeding esophageal varices, when he was through with one of these explosions of bleeding . . . was given a lot of steroids, and once he took off out of bed and out the window and a very small nurse . . . hung on to him. She was about five feet two inches, and he was six [feet] three [inches].[35]

While one nurse attended a patient with congestive heart failure who required rotating tourniquets, another patient with tetanus may have begun seizing; while a nurse reapplied silver nitrate bandages to a burned patient, another patient may have pulled out his chest tube. At some hospitals during the early 1950s, cardiac surgery patients came directly to the general wards from the operating room. These patients may have still been semiconscious and at risk for aspiration, shock, and hemorrhage. Dangers were intensified on the evening and night shifts, when nurse staffing traditionally reached its lowest point.

The 1950s became a critical period for questioning the traditional organization of nurses' work. Although functional, task-oriented care worked as a sort of control mechanism for busy nurses with limited skills, it proved a dangerous method of caring for the growing number of physiologically unstable patients in hospitals.

Traditional Assumptions About the Organization of Nurses' Work

In the 1950s, hospitals continued to cling to three traditional assumptions about nursing care: first, that hospitals should not bear the major costs of nursing care, to which end, they sought the cheapest care through the use of students and family-sponsored private-duty nurses; second, that decisions about the quality and quantity of nursing care were the domain of local hospitals, not national organizations; and third, that the nursing work force was unstable, transient, but constantly replenishable.

By relying on these assumptions about nursing care, hospitals found themselves with inexperienced nursing staffs unable to care for an increasingly complex hospital population. Hospitals' and nursing leaders' attempts to modify the care system, — by, for example, hiring less skilled care providers to extend the "hands and feet" of professional nurses — led only to diluted nursing staffs and even greater problems for the critically ill.

Historically, nursing students subsidized hospitals, which rapidly became labor-intensive, high-cash-flow businesses, through their unpaid student labor. During the 1950s, hospitals slowly moved away from the practice of student service, but it had not yet disappeared. Part of the reason for its longevity lay in the conflict between maintaining and increasing nursing services and keeping costs down in hospitals. Student service remained the most convenient, although not always the most cost-effective, method of reconciling the patient care conflict. For example, in 1946, the medical board of HUP noted that "a nurses' home [for both students and graduates] is far more important than the four extra floors [proposed for a new hospital building]. . . . This is essential for the proper functioning of the hospital."[36] This is a remarkable assessment of the value of students, in view of the potential for increased income that additional hospital rooms might have held for both the hospital and its physicians.

In contrast to hospitals' comfort with student labor, several influential surveys and reports of the 1940s and 1950s addressed the importance of skilled professional nursing care for all patients and deplored the use of students to staff hospitals. Many of these reports reaffirmed the emerging belief of nursing leaders that student service (unpaid student labor in hospitals) did not fit within either the goals of nursing education or the developing parameters of high-quality nursing care.[37] But as long as hospitals went unpenalized for determining their professional staffing needs by the number of students available for patient care, they resisted calls for predominantly professional nursing staffs.

Until the late 1950s, most students' weekly time schedules were based on the number of nurses needed to staff hospital units.[38] In 1957, the National League for Nursing reported that almost 70 percent of schools scheduled students' evening clinical experiences in this way. Only 43 percent of schools scheduled night experiences in advance. This meant that at times students were assigned to care for patients with problems for which the students had little classroom or practical preparation. These results led the NLN to conclude that, in a majority of instances, evening or night clinical experiences could "scarcely qualify as planned learning experiences but [are] more in the nature of work assignments."[39]

During their clinical assignments, students assumed tasks typically performed by both professional nurses and auxiliary workers.[40] Students easily approximated the work of auxiliary workers, but not that of graduate nurses. Like auxiliary workers, students required supervision. However, actual supervision by school instructors was marginal; supervision was provided primarily by hospital supervisors and head nurses.[41] While many nursing leaders supported the notion that one hundred student hours were the efficiency equivalent of seventy hours of professional care, many hospitals used students and professional nurses interchangeably, especially on evening and night shifts.[42]

Hospitals relied on their nursing schools not only for low-priced labor but also as a major supply pipeline for graduate nurse employment. During the 1950s, HUP annually employed 45 percent to 66 percent of the graduates of its nursing school, usually in September after August graduation.[43] In contrast, CHH employed from 58 percent to 100 percent of the graduating class per year, boosting the total number of professional nurses employed by 25 percent to 30 percent each September.[44] The hospital valued these nurses because they already were familiar with the hospital's way of doing things, were suitably loyal to the institution, and did not require orientation. Therefore, the value of the school lay both in the provision of cheaper nursing labor through the use of student service and in supplying a large pool of workers that easily and quickly merged into the hospital system.

The Costs of Nursing Care

At CHH in 1954 and 1955, students provided from 50 percent to 70 percent of the nursing care at the hospital.[45] The director of nursing estimated that the school saved the hospital more than $27,000 in labor costs in 1954. In 1950, when the amount of care provided by students probably exceeded 70 percent, the hospital earned a $3,900 profit from the school; student services were valued at $59,207.[46]

Financial problems plagued CHH, as they did many other small hospitals through the 1940s and 1950s; the hospital consistently ended these fiscal years with deficits or struggled through the year to end with small surpluses. During these years, a continuing dialogue took place among the board of trustees, the medical staff, and the nursing administration concerning the expense and responsibility of paying for nursing care.[47]

The concern of the trustees rested not only with nursing salaries but also with the indirect expenses associated with their increase. Nursing salaries appeared to be the benchmark for other nursing care personnel in the hospital. For example, in 1944 the trustees noted that a rise in graduate nursing salaries increased the cost of professional care to patients through both higher salaries for nurses and the resultant increases expected by other levels of workers.[48]

Nursing care costs attracted most of the board's criticism because they were a "new" and rapidly growing expense that hospital boards could no longer hide in institutional budgets or retrieve from patients' pockets. As nursing costs increased during the decade, so did costs for supplies such as food, medications, and utilities; however, hospitals had traditionally assumed the cost of these items and expected yearly increases. In 1952, expenses of the CHH's nursing department, although responsible for a large percentage of the hospital's rising costs, were lower than the Pennsylvania average. The proportion of expenses spent by the hospital for "operation of plant, repair, and upkeep" was higher than the state average, and the proportion spent for laboratory expenses exceeded the state average by almost 100 percent.[49]

For the first four fiscal months of 1947, the hospital faced a deficit of $21,000.[50] The trustees attributed their precarious financial situation to a decreased summer census and an increased cost of operations and noted that nursing salaries contributed the largest increase in expense. Accordingly, the trustees suggested that, because "nothing can be done about the increased rate of nursing salaries, this being a nationwide condition, it is essential that we bend every effort to increase enrollment in our training school, so we may take care of more of our nursing by students instead of registered nurses."[51]

The trustees had legitimate concerns about the cost of nursing care as nursing salaries increased 82 percent between 1944 and 1947. But they incorrectly located their problem in the amount of each nurse's salary, which they considered too high for women, rather than in the total amount of the nursing payroll. Only two salary increases occurred between 1944 and 1947, the second one followed by new and more favorable Blue Cross contract negotiations that gave the hospital almost $1.50 more per patient day (which more than covered the salary increase).[52] Later, a similar relationship emerged between nursing salaries and room rate increases.[53] This meant that the public still paid a portion of nursing care expenses in the form of higher insurance rates or out-of-pocket expenses, and the hospital continued to rely upon these sources to subsidize nursing care.

A report commissioned by the CHH trustees in 1944 (completed in 1948), during a bleak economic period for both the country and the hospital, further documented the hospital's reluctance to pay for professional nursing care and its attempts to define the care nurses provided according its own self-interest. The report, commissioned to identify ways to cut hospital expenses, noted that "the first department which deserves attention because of its marked increase in cost is the Nursing Department." [54]

The physician charged with preparing the report suggested that the reason for the increased expense of graduate nurses was high public expectations. He noted that the "public needs reeducation on this matter as, it also appears in some instances, does the physician." [55] To the report's author, hospital-financed nursing care consisted only of specific activities performed on physician orders. Personal, semispecial nursing of patients, or the "time-consuming refinements of nursing," should only be provided, he suggested, when the patient shares in the expense. [56] He subsequently recommended that the director of nursing reduce nursing care expenses by 25 percent through the use of less expensive workers and a greater number of students.

The hospital followed the report's suggestions and decreased its registered nurse population from sixty-one in November 1947 to fifty-four in February 1948, a 11.5 percent decrease over three months and a savings of $3,000. The committee noted that, when "a pinch of decreased numbers is felt, we can fill some of our nurse requirements by the use of 'Nurses Aides,' thus keeping up a proper standard of nursing, but at somewhat less cost." [57] Not surprisingly, the hospital noted a $3,500 surplus in April 1948. [58]

The director of both the school of nursing and the nursing service closely aligned herself with the hospital trustees and administrator on the matter of cost cutting. The finance committee praised the director, noting in 1952 that she had saved the hospital $12,000 in the past fiscal year. By doing so, however, the director had allowed the hours of nursing care per patient to drop to 2.6 per 24-hour period. [59] Although she noted two months later that "the nursing hours per patient were rather low," she reassured the board of trustees that "the situation will improve by the end of January when the students finish their courses at Temple [University]." [60] In 1940, Blanche Pfefferkorn had recommended an average of 4.7 hours of care per patient; in 1950, the Division of Nursing Resources of the U.S. Public Health Service suggested 3.5 hours. The nursing care staff at HUP provided an average of 3.1 hours of care in 1950. [61]

In December 1952, complaints about the shortage of nurses accelerated despite the fact that the hospital employed more nurses

than ever before. Two factors fueled the complaints: the time of
year and the greatly reduced number of admissions to the school
of nursing in 1950. In December, traditionally, a low number of
students were available for clinical work because the first-year students were scheduled for classes at Temple University until the end
of the month.[62] In 1950, the school of nursing admitted only twelve
first-year students (compared to twenty-four in 1949 and twenty-
three in 1951). This meant that the senior class, reaching a low of
only eight students in 1952, could not provide the usual boost in
nursing service expected from this advanced level of student.

The seeming contradiction between the increased numbers of
nurses hired by the hospital and complaints of nurse shortage is
also partially explained by rapidly changing work hours. Nurses
worked a forty-eight-hour week in 1950 and forty-four hours per
week in 1951. In February 1953, the board of trustees put into
effect a forty-hour work week for graduate nurses. The board did
not anticipate increased costs associated with filling a four-hour
deficit for each nurse on each shift because thirty-nine preclinical students were expected to be released for clinical duty shortly
before the change took place.[63] However, the thirty-nine students
did not completely fill the gaps created by the decreased number
of weekly graduate nurse hours, especially on the night shift. By
March 1953, the hospital increased the salary for graduate nurses
by ten dollars per month and increased the night premium from
ten to twenty dollars, to entice nurses to work the night shift.
Nurses responded to the financial incentive; the administrator reported that the hospital employed four additional nurses after initiating the raise.[64]

The hospital trustees were caught in a vicious cycle of their
own making. They complained about costs and attempted to reduce the nursing staff from October through February by not re-
placing nurses who resigned; but they discovered that adequate
nursing care could not be delivered with the pared-down staff, despite the release of students in February 1953 for clinical work.
In March 1953, the trustees renewed complaints about a nursing
shortage and raised salaries and premiums to attract new nurses
or pull nurses from other shifts to evenings and nights. In turn,
the board complained that nursing service contributed 50 percent
of the total budget increases in June 1953.[65] Caught in this self-
perpetuating cycle, the board could not claim financial relief from

the savings achieved by a smaller nursing staff, nor could it take comfort from the nursing shortage experienced by the hospital's patients.

Empowered Accreditation Agencies

The cycle of adjustment in professional nurse employment and expense containment continued in hospitals until the late 1950s, when an empowered accreditation body, the National League for Nursing, began to enforce nationally defined standards for quantity and quality of nursing care. Accreditation, or rather the threat of loss of it, became a powerful incentive for hospitals to look beyond their local communities to define acceptable standards of nursing care; local, traditional standards, usually based on economics rather than on the nursing care needs of patients, could no longer be used to design the education of student nurses or the nurse staffing needs of hospitals. A negative report, loss of accreditation, or only temporary accreditation with possibility of resurvey represented a major blow to any school of nursing. Presumably, decreased enrollments and loss of prestige would result. At HUP, changes in student utilization came in 1957 after the school of nursing received an unfavorable report from the NLN accreditation visit. The unfavorable report represented a harsh reality to a school many considered one of the best in Philadelphia and in the country.

Part of the NLN's criticism of the school involved the use of students for staffing purposes. In anticipation of the NLN visit and to gain some control over students' clinical schedules, the school attempted to initiate curriculum changes in 1956 and 1957. The school recognized the importance of aligning the philosophy and purpose of the school with the emerging educational trends presented in contemporary reports. But the school never formalized these plans; the NLN report noted, "It was not practical at this time in view of the need to maintain the constant flow of students to the nursing units of the hospital."[66] The report also pointed out that student clinical hours deviated considerably from the actual planned rotation program, with a greater number of clinical hours in practice than originally scheduled.[67]

The possibility of the loss of accreditation and, eventually, even of the school itself persuaded the hospital administration and the school overseers that the suggestions offered by an NLN consultation visitor were in their best interests.[68] The 1958 resurvey report documented the changes, noting: "It is now possible to estimate [the number of staff nurses needed] realistically, since the student nurse rotation schedules have been definitely established, in advance, by the faculty, school of nursing, and nursing service, [who] have planned jointly on the use of certain units for student experiences."[70]

Professional staffing of evening and night shifts improved by 1958, primarily through attempts by the school of nursing to gain accreditation. Because of the resultant decrease in the number of students on evening and night shifts, the hospital moved nurses and auxiliary workers to these shifts and hired more nurses for other shifts. The director of nursing service began to formalize shift plans in advance and gradually moved the hospital to a staffing system built around the graduate nurse rather than the student nurse.[71]

The total percentage of patient care given by professional nurses rose from less than 15 percent in the early 1950s[71] to approximately 45 percent in 1960. Night-shift staffing showed the greatest change: professional nurses provided only 16 percent of patient care on the night shift in 1957, compared to 50 percent in 1960. The percentage of care given by graduate nurses on the day shift, however, did not change drastically, due in part to the large increase in the percentage of care given by students and a 12 percent decrease in auxiliary-provided care.[72]

Overall, the changes signaled a breakdown in traditional assumptions. HUP quickly realized that, in terms of prestige or accreditation, using students as the primary caregiving labor force no longer paid and that local, parochial standards were not always appropriate benchmarks for nursing staffing or quality of care. The hospital grudgingly came to see the value of hiring more graduate nurses, if only to avoid loss of accreditation.

Patient-Financed Care: Private-Duty Nurses

In this transitional period, hospitals still relied on private patients' purchase of their own nursing care. Therefore, staffing for private, and to a lesser extent semiprivate, patients relied heavily on a ready cadre of private-duty nurses. Surgery might be canceled, despite the loss of income to the hospital and surgeon, if a private-duty nurse was unavailable. "Mr. C. will have to be covered [with a private-duty nurse]," the registrar's logbook at HUP noted, "or they will cancel his operation."[73]

Each private-duty nurse employed by a patient meant that hospitals' responsibility to provide, train, and pay nurses decreased by one. Between 1950 and 1960, the number of private-duty nurses employed by HUP paralleled 96 percent of its professional nursing force.[74] For example, in 1958, the hospital employed an average of 124 nurses; families employed an average of 119 private-duty nurses over the same time period.[75] This large-scale hiring of independent practitioners by families provided a "free" labor source that enabled hospitals to avoid other, more expensive strategies such as hiring more nurses.

As the complexity of the hospital population grew, so did the demand for private-duty nurses. Between 1950 and 1955, national demands for private-duty nurses increased faster than the number of private-duty nurses employed by patients in hospitals.[76] At HUP in 1954, patients submitted 8,409 requests for private-duty nurses, but 22.7 percent (1,909) of the requests went unfilled.[77] The comparable national rate for unfilled private-duty requests stood at 31 percent in 1955.[78]

Physicians at HUP complained about the unfilled requests, citing the twin culprits of nurses' loss of a sense of duty to the hospital and a shortage of staff and private-duty nurses. The problem proved to be more complex. There may have been enough nurses for each request to be filled, but private-duty nurses used their prerogative to refuse certain assignments or unpopular shifts.[79] In 1950, the medical board decided to increase the fee for evening-shift private-duty nurses by one dollar because of the large number of unfilled requests for private-duty nurses during that shift.[80]

One physician at another university hospital asserted, "These nurses . . . have little feeling of obligation to patients because they can, and do, sign off whenever they want to. 'Sorry, I can only work three days because the weekend is coming up.' So they leave. They feel no obligation to be on at all times."[81] Another view of the problem focused on a perceived shortage of "skilled" private-duty nurses. A physician at HUP noted, "We were running out of trained nurses. . . . You got to know who the good ones were, but you couldn't always get them. . . . There was a shortage of

ones that were really good."[82] Still another factor pointed to by
some was that private-duty nurses tended to be older women who
may not have "kept up" with the changes in medical care. For example, some private-duty nurses refused to care for "chest cases"
or patients recovering from cardiac surgery.[83] One private-duty
nurse removed herself from a case, noting, "This is a hard case
and [I am] unable to cope with it."[84]

Until the late 1950s, hospitals attempted to solve the problems
of increased labor costs by relying on traditional, inward-looking
practices of using student nurses and family-financed care. As a
result, the parameters of nursing care and the knowledge needed
to provide it remained situationally and locally defined until newly
powerful education and hospital-accreditation organizations man-
dated change.

An Unstable Work Force in an Unstable Environment

As hospitals began to lose access to traditional, homegrown sources
of cheap student labor or patient-financed nursing care, they were
confronted with a very fluid and temporary professional nurse
labor pool. High turnover, seasonal work cycles, and short-term
career tracks complicated the process of hiring larger cadres of
professional nurses. Hospitals attempted to cope with these problems by constantly hiring new nurses and cheaper, less-skilled
workers to fill the gaps. That hospitals never really did more to
address their employment problems presents an intriguing set of
questions that point to the probability that expectations of short-
term employment were shared by both nurses and hospitals.

The Revolving Door

Conceptualizing their nursing care problem as simply a lack of
personnel in an otherwise functional system, hospitals set about
hiring more workers of all types, using what Esther Lucile Brown
called the "hands and feet" solution.[85] The strategy, combined with
the newly emerging concept of team nursing, had three parts:
hiring more personnel on all levels, using lower-skilled employees
for some tasks in order to extend the availability of skilled nurses

to a larger group of patients, and matching a series of predictable tasks and skills to the educational level of the employee. Under this strategy, the percentage rise in national employment of graduate nurses and auxiliary workers during the fifties was higher than the percentage rise in number of beds, patient admissions, or average daily patient census.[86] One parameter, the total number of bedside nurses per one hundred patients in hospitals, increased by 46 percent between 1951 and 1959.[87] Hospitals hired nonprofessional personnel at an even greater rate. Between 1950 and 1956, the total number of nonprofessional workers per one hundred patients increased 71 percent.[88] The same trends for professional nurses can be seen during the fifties decade at CHH and HUP. Additionally, from 1939 to 1956, HUP hired 87 percent more nonprofessional personnel.[89]

Neither the solution nor the problem was simply one of numbers, however. Pouring more personnel into the system could not stop the flow out of the system. Although hospitals claimed that they could not hire enough nurses, they actually meant that they could not keep the nurses they hired. In 1955, the national turnover rate for professional nurses stood at 67 percent, compared to 40 percent for female factory workers.[90] This meant that hospitals always employed large proportions of inexperienced nurses to care for the growing number of physically unstable patients.

Neither HUP nor CHH were immune to the problem of turnover. Turnover rates of nursing personnel at CHH ranged from a high of 80 percent in 1956 to a low of 52 percent in 1958. Between 1954 and 1959, the hospital lost an average of 82 (both full- and part-time) nursing care personnel per year (with a low of 61 in 1954 and a high of 107 in 1956).[91] A 1956 administrator's report noted that 26 of the 51 full-time graduate nurses employed by the hospital resigned in that year.[92]

The median length of employment at HUP in 1954 for staff nurses was one year and three months. Head nurses and supervisors, the most experienced nursing employees, not surprisingly displayed greater employment longevity, four and a half years. Nurses' aides displayed the shortest term of employment, eight months.[93] By 1959, the median length of employment for staff nurses declined to approximately seven months; the median length of employment for head nurses and supervisors rested at four and a half and ten and a half years, respectively.[94]

More nurses left their staff nurse jobs for marriage and pregnancy than for any other single reason. A 1955–1956 survey from CHH revealed that more than half of the nurses who resigned cited marriage or pregnancy as the reason.[95] A study of four thousand Pennsylvania nurses pointed to the "strategic importance of children" and marriage in predicting work longevity.[96] A Missouri study indicated that 71 percent of nurses who resigned did so because of childbirth.[97]

Nurses graduating from training in the 1950s, however, were more likely than colleagues who had graduated in previous decades to return to work after marriage or while their children were young. The proportion of active nurses who were married increased from 46 percent to 61 percent between 1951 and 1962. Although nurses in the childbearing years (thirty-nine years or younger) represented the greatest proportion of inactive nurses, this proportion decreased from 67 percent in 1951 to 52 percent in 1962.[98] These nurses helped meet hospitals' constant need for nurses. Because many of those returning to the labor force after marriage or pregnancy were part-time workers, however, they could provide little continuity of care in a hospital environment that desperately needed a stabilizing force.[99]

Married nurses' return to the labor force reflected both women's role in supplementing the family's income and the changing roles of women in society.[100] In general, nurses followed national trends of the female nonfarm workforce. Between 1940 and 1960, the proportion of wives at work doubled, from 15 percent to 30 percent of the female labor force. The number of mothers at work increased 400 percent; mothers with children under eighteen were almost 30 percent of all women workers.[101] Although a 1954 study by Robert Bullock suggested that only 12 percent of the five hundred nurses surveyed planned to make a career of hospital nursing, 77 percent planned to return to nursing after marriage, but only to supplement their husband's income.[102] Regardless of why they returned to work at certain points in their lives, nurses expected to move back easily into the hospital system. Although salaries remained low and advancement difficult, nursing was one of the only professions guaranteeing jobs for women.

Despite the fact that hospitals complained about the shortage of nurses, administrators and nurses may have held shared expectations of short-term, cyclical employment.[103] This is a reasonable assumption in light of the advantages short-term employment offered to hospitals and nurses. Hospitals benefited because they could employ a large group of nurses at lower, entrance-level salaries. Nurses benefited through the flexibility offered by the numerous positions available and the ease with which they could return to work after raising a family. A president of the board of managers at HUP acknowledged the pluses of short-term employment, saying, "It's a little mystifying as to why hospital nursing isn't a more attractive career to young women when you think of the security nursing brings, not only in terms of work right after graduation but in bringing up a family and obtaining employment at any time."[104] A physician at the same hospital added, "I understand that nationally nursing school graduates work an average of only seven months on their first job. It's a peripheral benefit of course, but perhaps we should emphasize the excellent preparation that nurses's training provides for marriage and family life."[105]

Unmarried nurses anticipated similar flexibility, moving from job to job or taking vacations during the summer months. These nurses made active decisions to improve their work situations that took them beyond the grasp of traditional institutional loyalty or family responsibility. Such choices were possible because of the larger array of prospective jobs. Unlike nurses in training before the 1940s, nurses in the 1950s had options other than private duty. Staff nursing demand, other new positions in the hospital (such as operating room nursing), and positions outside the hospital (such as industrial nursing) made nurses' job movement easier and less risky. Nurses understood that positions in hospitals would always be available to them.[106]

Seasonality of Nurses' Employment

It is difficult to appraise the nursing workforce in hospitals because the number of nurses employed appears to have followed seasonal trends, as did complaints about the shortage of nurses.[107] Nurses' seasonal work trends were not a phenomenon limited to the 1950s and 1960s, but were traditional employment patterns of nurses. Mary Ross defined private-duty nursing in 1921 as "seasonal trade" because of the lower employment rates in the summer when the population was healthiest.[108] At HUP during the 1950s, the number of private-duty nurse requests decreased in the summer months because of the lower patient census. The percentage of filled requests also decreased as nurses chose not to work during the summer months.[109]

The number of nurses employed at HUP steadily decreased from a yearly high in September to a yearly low in August. In 1958, 48 percent of those who resigned did so from June to September. By March, the number of nurses employed at the hospital appeared, on the average, to be two-thirds lower than the September figure.[110] A similar seasonal flow and ebb of nurse employment is also seen at CHH.[111]

The cyclical nature of the number of nurses employed at the two hospitals may be attributed to several factors. Hospitals employed a large number of nurses after September graduations. Newly graduated nurses occasionally worked from September until April or May and then resigned in order to travel. In 1958, 8 percent of those who resigned from HUP did so "to travel" to destinations such as Europe, Colorado, or Hawaii. After their travels, they returned to full-time employment.[112] At certain times of the year, hospitals may not have replaced those who resigned. As a hospital approached the end of the fiscal year (from March to May), especially if it was operating with a deficit and a low patient census, hiring of new nurses may have been put off until September when the census traditionally increased and the budget appeared more flexible.[113]

Net Loss of Skills

Along with hiring more personnel overall, the "hands and feet" solution involved two additional components: first, hiring less-skilled employees to extend the skills of nurses to a larger group of patients and, second, matching a series of predictable tasks and skills to the educational level of the employee. Lambertsen's concept of team nursing, proposed as a philosophy of nursing care and communication, offers one such example of how the solution should have operated.[114] Team nursing, as intended by Lambertsen, "expanded" the skills of the professional nurse by putting her in charge of a number of less skilled workers to care for a group of patients.

Hospitals, however, co-opted the team concept because it made economic sense and was familiar; team nursing resembled the successful system of volunteer aides and orderlies used during World War II. Instead of relying on the concept's original intent as an organizational philosophy to restructure nurses' work around the needs of the patient, hospitals exploited the concept as an administrative strategy to structure tasks around the abilities of less expensive workers. By changing the focus of work from the patient to the worker, hospitals gained a cheap method of providing nursing care. Patients, in turn, lost access to a professional nurse and were confronted with workers with fewer skills.

Inappropriate use of workers magnified the problems of team nursing and exaggerated the changes occurring in hospitals. First, hospitals of the 1950s attempted to build a care system that required stable environments and a predictable series of routine tasks—in an environment that was not stable or predictable. Hospitals of the 1950s were in transition from units full of convalescent patients to units full of severely ill, physically unstable, and chronically ill people (see Chapter 2). Team nursing may have worked for general obstetrics, pediatrics, or rehabilitation units, but when modestly prepared nurses were confronted with the addition of even one critically ill patient, chaos resulted. The already fluid boundaries between levels of workers broke down; those with less skill were called upon to perform tasks for which they were untrained. Professional nurses assumed nonnursing tasks themselves rather than rely upon the auxiliary team members.[115]

Fluidity of the boundaries of professional nursing care served to intensify conflicts between professional nurses and auxiliary workers, especially practical nurses. Professional nurses saw practical nurses encroaching upon their newly established position in hospitals, especially when the parameters of nursing care were not clearly defined and were open to situational interpretation. Registered nurses resented practical nurses' taking for themselves the cherished symbols of professional nurses—the cap and the pin. Nurses should fear usurpation, wrote one nurse, because most patients "knew little about the distinction in responsibilities and abilities."[116] In Philadelphia, the conflict did not appear to be as pronounced as elsewhere due to the large number of registered nursing schools in the city, where the professional nurse maintained a monopoly until the late 1950s.[117] Nationally, however, the conflict raged, as exemplified by the exchange of letters in national journals. One nurse noted in 1952, "I understood that the Journal was for [registered nurses]. Let's keep it that way. . . . They [practical nurses] have taken our caps and pins. . . . Must we give them our journal too?" A reply to this author more astutely addressed the dangers of less educated workers: "I would sleep better at night if I knew they [practical nurses] had it and read it."[118]

The above reply helps to articulate the second problem inherent in team nursing: nurses found themselves responsible for workers who did not know a lot, and many nurses themselves did not have the skills needed for team supervision or the care of physically unstable patients. Auxiliary workers could not work unsupervised, nor could they initiate action during an emergency, such as administering a sedative to an agitated patient or determining when the patient in fulminating congestive heart failure required rotating tourniquets. A glaring and dangerous discrepancy existed between the characteristics of the staff and the problems presented by a growing population of physically unstable patients.

William H. Stuart, former surgeon general of the United States, summed up the problem, noting that "when you expand your personnel pyramid with nurses at the top you have more and more, lesser and lesser trained people making up that pyramid. . . . [That which was] designed to extend the hands and skills of this professional nurse actually ends up in defeating its purpose. The result is a net loss rather than a gain."[119]

Conclusion

After World War II, nursing moved from an independent, patient-centered, private-duty practice to an institutional, bureaucratic practice in hospitals. Nursing was unprepared for the transition. Nurses lacked the skills, education, and authority needed to care for groups of patients who were progressively physically unstable in an environment that was constantly growing in size and complexity. Attempts to address the skills and knowledge deficit met with trouble because no one really knew exactly what nurses should be able to do in the hospitals of the 1950s. This was dramatically documented by the more than forty attempts to define the work of nurses through nursing function studies and the wide range of study results.

The diverse opinions about nurses' work resulted in two very different coping strategies. One strategy sought national nursing education reform. An empowered training school and hospital accreditation process began to differentiate nursing education from nursing practice, thus allowing education to evolve independently of hospital staffing needs. This measure substantially shaped nursing education into a more contemporary model and was the product of concerned nursing leaders.

The second strategy was local, grassroots problem-solving driven by the self-interests and particular experiences of hospitals as each attempted to resolve the conflict between the need for professional nursing care and economic concerns. Parochial problem-solving ensured that each training school and hospital developed its own definition of "good" nursing care. Nevertheless, hospitals nearly simultaneously stumbled onto the intensive care solution.

The limits of the second strategy became obvious in the early intensive care units. Critically ill patients required nurses with the skills and knowledge to take action rather than inexperienced, functionally educated caretakers. Nurses caring for critically ill patients had to have the knowledge and expertise to make clinical decisions. No formal system helped nurses acquire the needed knowledge or delineated what they needed to know; a giant chasm existed between the nursing education reform ideas of national nursing leaders, who were logically concerned with separation of education and practice, and the practices of nurses in local hospitals, who saw nursing as functionally driven, temporary employment with flexible boundaries.

Chapter 4
Negotiating New Roles

One of the defining characteristics of the new intensive care units of the 1950s and 1960s was the way doctors and nurses allocated the work of patient care. Because of factors such as the architecture of the new units, the inexperience of both physicians and nurses, and a realization by physicians that nurses had to have greater authority over patient care decisions, nurses and physicians redefined the way they worked together, what the work was, and who had the responsibility and authority for certain tasks. Through deal-making, collaboration, trading off, or informally reaching agreements, nurses took on responsibilities of patient care in the hospitals of the 1950s and 1960s that complemented and enhanced the ongoing reform of nursing care and nursing education.

Traditional Relationships

The relationship between nurses and physicians and the division of the work of patient care was always negotiated against a backdrop of social, economic, political, and gender constraints that limited nurses' authority in patient care decisions.[1] After trained nurses entered hospitals in the late nineteenth century, lay trustees delegated power to the nurse (the superintendent or matron) to manage the hospital. Physicians, practicing primarily outside of the hospital, held little line authority over the nurse superintendent. Later, however, as hospitals became more acceptable places for the middle and upper classes to recover from illness, and in particular to undergo surgery, medical practice became more and more hospital based and associated with the financial success of the hospital through physician-generated admissions.[2] Lay trustees became less interested in daily hospital operations and physicians became more powerful in hospital management, usurping the authority of the matrons or superintendents. Nurses' lack of power made them dependent on physicians for clinical authority, especially since nurses had less formal education (secondary education versus collegiate education), were in general from lower social classes, and lacked the means to bring income to the hospital. All in all, nurses lost parity with physicians in negotiating patient care responsibilities.[3]

Barbara Melosh argues that nurse migration from private-duty practice to institutional nursing in the 1940s gave nurses "protection by structure" from dependent economic and work relationships with physicians. Protection by structure, in Melosh's analysis, included more favorable salary structures, work environments, and job policies in which work was determined by hospital supervisors rather than by patients and physicians.[4] We argue, however, that the movement of nurses into hospitals failed to gain greater authority or power for nurses over the division of patient care work. Although physicians, in fact, controlled private-duty nurse participation in some registries and patients dictated some structure, private-duty nurses held considerable autonomy and authority over their practice. Private-duty nurses could choose the assignments and shifts they desired. Once employed, private-duty nurses worked on their own. Physicians were distanced from the practice setting of the home.[5]

If there was actually any protection by structure as nurses moved their practice to hospitals, the protection proved fairly superficial and repressive. Nurses lost a great deal of autonomy and independence in the paternalistic authority structure of hospital employment. In the hospital, physicians controlled nurses in two important ways: by wielding authority both over nursing care and over the nurses themselves. Physicians manifested control through their roles as lecturers and trustees in nurse training schools and as the conduit for nurses' clinical authority.[6] The "captain of the ship" metaphor characterized nurse-physician interactions and was manifested in various behaviors and rituals to remind both parties of the hospital hierarchy. "A tactful nurse," wrote the editor of a charity society newsletter in 1903, "will preserve to some extent the fiction of working under the physician's direction; and those who can guide and prevent stupid blunders, and even prevent positive injuries, while still appearing to follow and to obey instructions, represent perhaps the flower of the nursing profession."[7]

Until the 1950s, there were too few nurses to make any real difference in the negotiation of work parameters—hospitals relied on transient and cheap student labor for patient care. Until this time, most nurses hired by hospitals worked in administrative positions such as head nurse or supervisor rather than in clinical positions where the informal negotiations about patient care took place. Nurses who were functioning at some distance from direct patient care gained little from renegotiated practice, even though the patient population's care needs became more complex. Nor was negotiation a political reality for students socialized to the importance of loyalty to the physician as an essential component of a patient's therapy.[8]

In a confusing twist, social behaviors in the hospital were opposite those expected in public. Even as late as the 1950s, female nurses and students were expected to rise when male physicians entered a room, or to carry heavy loads of charts while physicians made rounds unencumbered. Nurses were also expected to offer their chairs to the physician.[9] Paradoxically, physicians unofficially relied upon nurses to police medical practice; physicians assumed nurses would remind them when medical orders needed rewriting or a break in sterile technique occurred.[10] For example, the highest priority for a new isolation unit at Hospital of the University of Pennsylvania (HUP) was "a firm administrative head nurse" who could keep physicians in line.[11] At Chestnut Hill Hospital (CHH), supervisors instructed nurses in the operating room to enforce the rules of the infection control committee, including reporting physicians to the director of nursing. Later attempts to enforce the standards stipulated by the medical staff resulted in "ill feelings and ill will, discourteous treatment, frequently over the telephone, from some physicians. . . . They feel as nurses and as ladies, they are unable to enforce these regulations."[12]

As hospitals employed more graduate nurses to provide direct patient care, nurses began to use certain rituals and behaviors to subtly display their expertise while supporting physicians' traditional place in the hierarchy. The "doctor-nurse game" described by Leonard Stein in 1967 outlined the classic example of such behaviors. The object of the game for nurses was to impart valuable information to the physician about the patient's case, displaying the expertise of the nurse but allowing patient care decisions to appear to be based on physician-generated information.[13] A nurse, for example, might ask, "Dr. Brown, what do you think about the patient's color?" To which the physician might reply, "The patient is a little blue—I'm going to order oxygen. Nurse, please start oxygen." Nursing school leaders also participated in the game by socializing their pupils to be loyal and obedient to physicians; nurses were taught that if they failed to do so they risked losing what little authority they had.

The nurses working in the hospitals of the late 1940s and early 1950s were primarily young, newly graduated nurses. They lacked the "history" of autonomous and entrepreneurial practice of the private-duty nurse and followed the "the physician is the undisputed leader of patient care" mantra propagated by their nursing instructors, physician lecturers, and society at large. Only dangerous situations and opportunities for showcasing their expertise would provide nurses with the impetus to overcome the effects of socialization. Then, frustrated staff nurses sought out solutions with like-minded physicians, but with little help from preoccupied nursing leaders. These individual and small-group responses were local and parochial in nature, but they represented a groundswell of grassroots patient care reform.

Renegotiating Care

As the patient population of hospitals grew more complex in the 1950s, an overextended nursing and medical staff tried to keep their patients safe. Patient mortality and morbidity due to a lack of successful therapy was an unfortunate circumstance. In fact, thre was always a sense of uncertainty about outcomes in medical practice.[14] But when patients died because nurses and physicians were too busy to observe respiratory distress or hemorrhage, or because they didn't know what to do about such common crises, all parties took notice. Nurses and physicians caring for these patients discussed their fears and looked for solutions.

One of the informal solutions was situational credentialing (giving nurses the unspoken authority to respond to particular patient care situations). When their most helpless patients were at risk, nurses and physicians temporarily discarded traditional patterns of communication and behavior. For example, nurses may have had the authority to diagnose a patient's problem and initiate treatment at night when a physician was unavailable. "Whatever I did I let the doctor know," one nurse noted. "I was there, he wasn't, and sometimes decisions had to be made right then. If you found the physician it might be too late. . . . I didn't want to lose the patient."[15] Once a physician arrived on the scene, the nurse returned authority for her actions to the physician. This process of situational credentialing allowed quick patient treatment without the physician's loss of authority.

By nature, this informal transfer of authority based on contingency was inconsistent and dangerous. Gaining authority to perform work according to circumstance is a fluid concept dependent upon the "desires, aspirations, energies, and goals" of the person allocating permission.[16] For example, a nurse had to understand which physicians allowed overstepping of traditional task boundaries. Would Dr. Smith overlook the nurse's venture into medical territory, or would he report her actions to the supervisor? Each nurse had to undertake her own time-consuming negotiation with individual physicians.[17] As part of the negotiation process, each nurse had to certify her wealth of skills to each physician. Nurses had to earn acknowledgment of their competence. In contrast, physician expertise was assumed until proven otherwise.[18] Although these assumptions gradually changed as nursing education reforms took place in the 1960s and 1970s, nurses still spent valuable time proving their expertise.

When physicians and nurses could not productively resolve the overlapping boundaries of skill and authority, work conditions deteriorated for both parties. Controlling and withholding information was a powerful tool used by both nurses and physicians when negotiations did not work. For example, physicians might withhold records from nurses or fail to teach nurses about the proper use of equipment. On the other hand, nurses might use their knowledge of hospital rules to frustrate physicians by refusing to honor verbal rather than written orders.[19] Patients suffered when nurses and physicians failed to cooperate.

When physicians instigated new types of treatments or therapies without negotiating responsibilities with nurses, failure sometimes followed. For example, Hugh Day, a cardiologist at Bethany

Hospital in Kansas City, Kansas, had concerns about high coronary mortality rates, which prompted him to develop the "Hirsch Crash Cart." He introduced the cart on the general wards for ten months in the early 1960s, but saw no improvement in mortality rates. The hospital had too few nurses to keep a close watch on the cardiac patients, and patients experienced difficulties long before they were found by the nurses. Additionally, the nurses did not know what to do once the patient was found in distress. Because of nurse staffing shortages and high turnover, few nurses received instruction on the emergency care of these patients or on how to use the equipment and medications on the crash cart.[20] Similarly, when Dr. Day introduced cardiac monitors on the general floor, no one taught the nurses about arrhythmias or how to turn off the monitor alarms. Nurses, feeling left out of the process and unable to respond, began to call the physicians at all hours of the day and night when the alarms sounded. Shortly thereafter the monitors were removed from the general floors, and in 1962 the hospital established a separate coronary care unit with centralized monitors and a more knowledgeable staff.[21]

When successful negotiations occurred, nurses and physicians created enterprising solutions to patient care problems. All across the country, nurses and physicians came together to devise strategies for caring for critically ill patients. At CHH in 1954, a shortage of residents, interns, and private-duty nurses (who usually cared for the critically ill at the family's expense) compelled Dr. William McClenahan, an internist, to suggest a separate area staffed with expert nurses to care for critically ill patients. But costs concerned the hospital trustees who anticipated a year-end budget deficit and estimated that the extra nurses to staff the unit would cost the hospital $1,800 per month.[22]

Dr. McClenahan then discussed the matter with the hospital administrator and the director of nursing. Both realized that critically ill patients benefited from easy observation and concentrated nursing care; they also realized that the hospital did not want to absorb the cost and that the cost could not be transferred to private insurers.[23] The hospital's contract with the local Blue Cross organization explicitly stated that all nursing service had to be provided to patients without additional charge except for private-duty nursing, which was the responsibility of the subscriber.[24]

Private-duty nurses directly billed insured patients. Private-duty nurses also provided care to groups of patients; in fact, CHH encouraged this practice. The three problem solvers asked themselves, "Why couldn't the hospital do the same? Wouldn't two to three nurses caring for six patients constitute a simple form of group private-duty nursing?"[25]

To obtain Blue Cross permission for the group nursing scheme, which was needed to avoid invalidation of the hospital contract, the administrator contacted the executive director of the Associated Hospital Services of Philadelphia, who was also a personal friend.[26] The director agreed to support the plan on an experimental basis and only at CHH. He insisted that Blue Cross's support remain "unannounced" because he feared a rapid surge in the use of these services and their eventual inclusion in the insurance contract.[27]

The only differences between CHH's private-duty arrangement at the time and the proposed solution was the party responsible for the billing and the cut-rate fee the hospital proposed to offer. Twenty-four-hour private-duty nursing cost patients and their families thirty-six dollars in 1954. The hospital proposed charging patients only twelve dollars for twenty-four-hour care in the new unit.[28] Once the group persuaded the hospital trustees and the insurer of the necessity of this ingenious solution, the special care unit opened a few months later in May 1954.

Grassroots negotiations concerning the care of the critically ill drew on the experiences of practicing nurses and physicians rather than already established policies of the hospital bureaucracy. Logically, this is the only way such bargaining could have taken place productively. As nurses and physicians tested new boundaries, debate could produce either expansion or contraction of boundaries; this process required an almost constant dialogue between care providers. Although national in scope, the problems of caring for increasingly complex patient populations could be addressed only by those caregivers intimately involved; the conception and execution of a new way of caring for critically ill patients took place in doorway conferences and backdoor maneuvering in local hospitals. Success depended upon the ability of nurses and physicians to negotiate the boundaries of patient care within the context of their own political and social means.

Why did nurses and physicians enter into negotiations transcending traditional divisions of work? What factors encouraged physicians, traditionally reluctant to relinquish authority over any elements of their practice, to share authority with nurses for crucial decision-making about the care of critically ill patients? And why did nurses, unskilled in the care of the critically ill and already overworked, accept, expand, and seek out broadened authority? We look at the relationships between physicians and nurses in early intensive care units to see how they defined, negotiated, and tested the division of the work of patient care over time.

The boundaries of the work of caring for patients in hospitals traditionally were negotiated within the context of ideology, politics, class, economics, and gender. It is important to recognize that negotiations of work boundaries first took place at the local level, in small, intimate settings such as recovery rooms, operating rooms, and intensive care units. Within these settings, closeness of quarters, familiarity between doctors and nurses, and experience (nurses' intimate knowledge of patients) helped bridge the discrepancies in knowledge and class.

These settings provided an ideal environment for testing a new model of nursing care based on patient stability. Usually placed in small areas such as unused closets or corners, the early ICUs supported experimentation and informal deal-making, trades of knowledge, and task realignments. The results of these local negotiations, such as enlarged responsibilities and authority for nurses or other patient care strategies, could be easily and immediately tested, promoted, renegotiated, or discarded without the oversight of formal hospital authorities or interference from professional organizations.

The new settings for care also invited physicians, albeit influenced by geography and situations at hand, to discard traditional assumptions gained through professional socialization and education about the expertise and abilities of nurses. This new way of thinking was in part facilitated by the overwhelming presence of graduate nurses rather than students in the units and by the increased complexity of the patient population. Acknowledging the complexity of care, nursing supervisors tended to assign their most experienced and knowledgeable graduate nurses to the intensive care units. By virtue of their concentration in a small area and their experience and knowledge, these nurses provided stability and reassurance to physicians and patients. Traditional socialization patterns were more easily breached when physicians realized the advantages and had both the courage and the opportunity to work with nurses in a less authoritative and self-conscious manner. Although cooperation between nurses and physicians in the rest of the hospital continued to be undermined by traditional social attitudes, the intensive care units served as a testing ground on which a more collaborative structure was explored and found to be beneficial.

Zones of Security, Authority, and Safety

The early intensive care units are an ideal microcosm for examining the fluid work boundaries between doctors and nurses in the complex hospital environment of the 1950s and 1960s (see Chapter 2). The units provided a "zone of security" for physicians worried about their critically ill patients. Physicians were not always available during emergencies and were sometimes unskilled in the care of physically unstable patients. As medical and technical therapies increased in complexity, many physicians could not keep up with medical advances, nor did they have time to personally monitor complex therapies.

For this zone of security to be realized, physicians had to acknowledge a partnership with nurses. In turn, nurses providing care for unstable patients needed the expertise, skills, and authority traditionally considered the domain and privilege of physicians. This included nurses' assessing the physical stability of patients and, in the absence of physicians, making critical decisions and treating patients according to protocols, without explicit, individualized physicians' orders.

Nurses gained a "zone of authority" to act within a sphere of competence in which their skills and expertise were respected and assumed. With authority, however, came the responsibility to learn more about the care of physically unstable patients. Expertise in this area required skills not taught in the usual training school curriculum but learned from self-education, experience, and physician teachers. Assuming these responsibilities put critical care nurses at risk of alienation from the broader corps of professional nurses. As professional nursing had abandoned nurse anesthetists in the 1940s and 1950s, so too would many early critical care nurses experience deliberate distancing by both local nursing authorities and professional nursing.[29]

For patients, the intensive care units provided a "zone of safety." Instead of working alone, caregivers pooled their knowledge about the care of critically ill patients. Established protocols, concentrated nursing and physician presence, shared knowledge, and rapid responses to changing patient stability gave critically ill patients greater protection in an uncertain hospital environment. Fewer diverging interests and less competitive strain allowed nurses and physicians to concentrate their time and energy on the care of the critically ill.[30]

The Physicians

The increasing complexity of patients of the 1950s required more intensive attention from physicians. However, physicians, many of whom had externally located office-based practices, spent a great deal of time outside of the hospital. This was particularly true of physicians practicing in community hospitals. In order to staff the hospital and provide medical coverage for patients at night, community hospitals and their physicians relied upon medical students, residents, and interns. But many community hospitals had difficulty recruiting the needed complement of interns and residents. For example, CHH desired a complement of five residents and five interns, but consistently failed to attract this number. In 1952, the administration noted, "We are having difficulty getting residents; four are leaving for various reasons on January 1, and we have only two to replace them."[31] "We are disappointed," noted the administrator in 1954. "The hospital has obtained only one internship for 1954–1955, we need five."[32]

Hospitals implemented creative solutions, such as utilizing foreign physicians when they failed to attract U.S. medical graduates. "The present interns are overworked, and we have received no answers from the U.S. and Canada," the medical staff committee at CHH reported, "but [have received] inquiries from men in Cyprus, Greece, and England. They are eager to come if they can get on the quota."[33] Although the hospital and medical staff welcomed these physicians, problems of language and culture sometimes limited their contributions.[34]

In the face of an intern or resident shortage, the only medical coverage at some community hospitals at night was the emergency room physician (or medical students hired to work in the emergency room) or the house physician (usually an intern or resident). During times of inadequate intern and resident coverage, staff physicians reluctantly took on the extra work. In September 1951, the staff at CHH decided that each physician had to serve as "officer of the day" on a rotating basis, but they discontinued the practice three months later because it was "too much of a burden."[35]

In an environment of thin medical coverage, physicians could not guarantee the survival of their physically unstable patients. Unstable patients required immediate treatment and could not wait for a physician to come from home or office. A patient in fulminating pulmonary edema required rapid decisions and treatments. Similarly, patients experiencing cardiac arrest had to be treated within four minutes to forestall cerebral anoxia.[36]

Physicians could not protect their patients themselves and, because hospitals were reluctant to take on the extra expense of physician coverage, had little choice but to cede certain decision-making responsibilities to nurses. The idea of hospital-based, salaried physicians, just becoming a reality in large university hospitals, was practically nonexistent in community hospitals.[37] Nurses were at hand and, for the most part, willing to do the work.

Physicians had to rely upon nurses both to diagnose the patient's problem and then to describe the scenario accurately to the physician over the phone. Eventually physicians also ceded certain essential treatment decisions to nurses. For example, nurses at Presbyterian Hospital Coronary Care Unit in Philadelphia could make the decision to defibrillate a patient before discussing the case with the physician.[38] Sharing of responsibilities for diagnosis and treatment, two of the pillars of medical therapeutics, became more common during emergency situations.

Although sharing diagnosis and treatment decisions represented landmark concessions by physicians to nurses, physicians really did not lose anything, nor was their professional dominance threatened. Physicians still held on to the "symbolic work" of devising protocols and writing orders, tasks that nurses were legally prevented from doing but were technically able to accomplish.[39] By sharing decision-making, physicians yielded some level of responsibility and conceded the expertise of nurses without relinquishing any real power or control. Nurses gained only uncodified authority in physicians' absence. In many situations, nurses still had to obtain post facto coverage for their actions through written

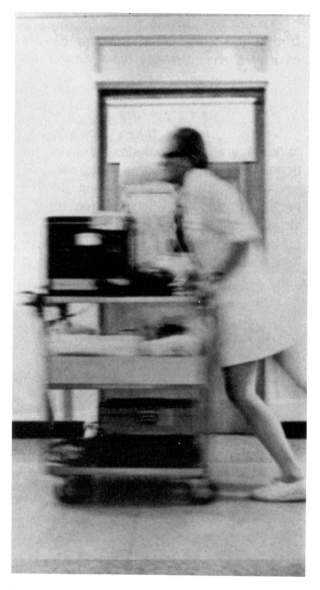

Figure 9. Nurse rushing to an emergency, circa 1970. From *Planning for Cardiac Care: A Guide to the Planning and Design of Cardiac Care Facilities* (Chicago: Health Administration Press, 1973), 71. Used with permission.

physician orders. In many hospitals and intensive care units, protocols guided nurses' responses to patient emergencies. Protocols allowed nurses to decide independently when certain treatments could be initiated, but they were tools to be used in a physician's absence.

Prescribed protocols strictly limited the scope of nurses' patient care decisions. They supported decision-making nonetheless, and their use represented an enormous change in working relationships of nurses and physicians.[40] When protocols did not exist, nurses and physicians continued to make informal contracts defining expanded boundaries of nurses' authority and responsibility. Without protocols, nurses had greater latitude for decision-making but made these decisions without legal protection. For example, in the early 1960s when closed-chest cardiac massage became an accepted form of treatment for cardiac arrest, information about the treatment filtered down from physicians to nurses. Nurses learned about the process informally, on an individual basis, and used closed-chest massage only when a tacit understanding with individual physicians provided security from disciplinary action. In the early 1960s, closed-chest massage was not considered within the authority and purview of nurses. Both the American Heart Association and the American Nurses Association (ANA) recommended that nurses only assist physicians during closed-chest massage, rather than initiate the procedure. The ANA took this stand in 1962 because the organization felt that nurses already took on too many tasks previously performed by physicians, the professional and legal implications were unclear, and, most importantly, nurses were unprepared to do the procedure.[41] The ANA changed its stand in 1965 because more evidence existed that the procedure worked and standards for performing and learning the procedure had been established by the American Heart Association.[42]

Early on, physicians realized that nurses should be prepared to do closed-chest resuscitation in the absence of a physician, as the procedure had to be started within four minutes of a cardiac arrest to prevent complications. If the arrest occurred at night, the possibility of physicians' arriving within that time frame was remote. The physicians at HUP debated formally allowing nurses to perform closed-chest cardiac massage. Because no agreement could be reached about nurses' role, the committee decided that "special instructions" from each physician to the nurses would be continued as before. Nurses at this hospital continued to perform closed-chest massage routinely, in the absence of physicians, without legal protection.[43]

Physicians risked less threat to their professional autonomy and power when they ceded responsibility informally. No evidence existed that any task or authority had indeed been shared. It was more difficult for nurses in general to expand their decision-making authority on an episode-by-episode basis. Informal contracts made by individuals at local hospitals were difficult to transfer to a national policy.

During the 1960s and 1970s, physicians and nurses experimented with expanding boundaries of responsibility and authority for nurses. Naturally, most of these experiments took place in isolated, local settings and involved perhaps one doctor and one nurse who developed a trusting relationship. These conditions provided "an opportunistic environment" for testing models.[44] In primary care settings, nurse practitioners and physician colleagues experimented with a new patient care delivery system predicated on nurses' expansion of boundaries into diagnosis and treatment. Rose Pinneo and Lawrence Meltzer at Presbyterian Hospital, Philadelphia, and Loretta Ford and Henry Silver collaborating in Colorado are just two examples of nurse-physician alliances formed during this period of changing relationships.

Certainly the formation of these alliances was helped along by the changes occurring in society at large, such as the women's movement and the civil rights movement. Linda Aiken and David Mechanic point to physicians' realization that their ability to remain "technically expert while providing humane care to patients depends upon the negotiated relationship with other health professionals, particularly nurses."[45] Stein and his colleagues cite the deterioration of public esteem for physicians, rising numbers of women in the medical profession, and a nursing shortage to explain changes in negotiation tactics. As they note, nurses "stopped playing the game."[46] Nurses were also better educated and more able to take on expanding responsibilities. Experiences from early intensive care units showed nurses needed more in-depth knowledge, including pathophysiology and psychosocial assessment skills. By the 1970s, many more nurses began to receive their education in liberal-arts-based collegiate baccalaureate programs where these concepts were part of the curriculum.

Even as individual nurses and physicians found common ground for more collegial relationships, "tensions at the bedside," present since the origins of organized nursing, perpetuated competition for control of bedside care and impeded sharing of the relationship with the patient.[47] Attempts by national organizations such as the American Medical Association (AMA) to initiate the registered care technician program and obstruct third-party payment for nurses reflected both economic tensions and fears about loss of control at the bedside.[48] In contrast, the National Joint Practice Commission, founded by the AMA and the ANA in 1971, was a major national effort to examine nurse-physician interactions through various models of care delivery.[49] Whether or not nurses and physicians moved on to higher and more generalized levels of collaboration depended upon resolution of tensions or barriers such as educational and social class differences, jurisdiction, and sex-role stereotypes.[50] Paradoxically, areas such as intensive care units invited local initiatives for greater collaboration but also magnified possibilities for even broader role negotiations. While the intensive care unit provided protection for patients of busy physicians, it also magnified the dysfunction created by physicians' sole control over patient care in the presence of expert nurses.

The Nurses

As hospital administrations ceded authority to nurses and physicians to devise new patient care models, a new level of work was created in the hospital hierarchy. An essentially grassroots movement took place out of reach of the hospital bureaucracy as nurses and physicians informally negotiated, through trial and error, new boundaries in patient care. Since the intensive care setting was a new concept, almost every boundary had to be reestablished and normalized. The negotiation process increased in complexity as boundaries were evaluated and renegotiated.

To gain expertise about the care of complex patients, nurses learned through experience and from physicians. Although many physicians were equally unskilled in the care of physically unstable patients, physicians provided much of nurses' postgraduate education through formal lectures and informal conversations. Nurses learned during slow periods in the intensive care area. During these times, residents (usually) and nurses in the intensive care unit discussed patients in detail, each learning from the other. When cardiac monitors were introduced at one hospital, a nurse remembered nurses and physicians grouped informally around the monitor screen in "pick-up" sessions. She noted that both physicians and nurses spent a lot of time looking at the monitor, recognizing that a rhythm looked different than normal and then paging through a manual or sample strips trying to compare patterns.[51] "I learned from being in the unit," another nurse remembered, "asking questions and working with physicians."[52] Unusually close camaraderie developed between nurses and physicians in the units because of the small areas, shared sense of adventure in the new setting, and the selection of the "expert nurses," usually young and "energetic," to staff the unit. "We [nurses and physicians] were all in this together," one nurse noted. We all learned from each other."[53]

The intense needs of acutely ill patients supported closer relationships between physicians and nurses as they learned together. "We had different relationships with physicians. People were sick and we worked side by side keeping them alive. We worked long hours and we didn't go home. Physicians appreciated what we knew and what we could do."[54] Emotional and geographic closeness, in turn, supported informal knowledge "trades." Nurses' strategic position at the patient's bedside enabled them to trade knowledge of the patient's condition for physician's knowledge of physiology or interpretation of data. Nurses also traded their own skills and knowledge (for example, how to gain cooperation from an angry patient or family, or data derived from their intuitive skills) for the physician's knowledge. Nurses made informal "deals" and performed favors for physicians to gain knowledge to complement their proof of expertise.[55]

Nurses in the units gained status and informal certification of expertise by accumulating knowledge and skills belonging to the higher status medical profession. In a way, nurses hitched a ride to the bargaining arena on the power of physicians. "We used his power," a nurse reflected about her relationship with a particular surgeon and his assistance in gaining better staffing from a reluctant nursing director.[56] Although nurses' position relative to physi-

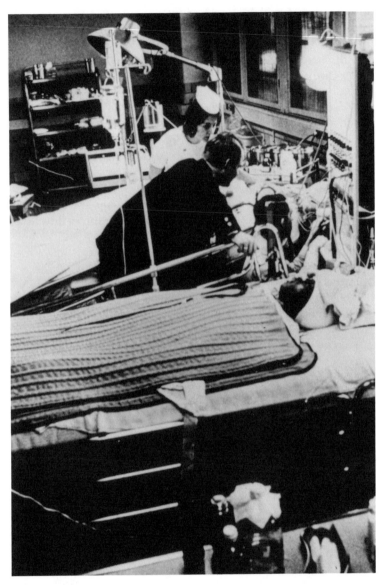

Figure 10. Nurse and physicians conferring about patient care, Philadelphia General Hospital, circa 1970. Courtesy of the Center for the Study of the History of Nursing, School of Nursing, University of Pennsylvania, Philadelphia, Pa.

cians did not change within the hospital hierarchy, nurses in the special care area acquired a distinctly different status from that of general floor nurses. Hospitals chose their "expert" nurses to work in the special care unit.[57] This implied to the rest of the nursing staff that these nurses were different from and better than those "left behind." Although most nurses in the special care areas did not admit to difficulties with other nurses, one gets the sense that most considered themselves to have been performing at a higher level. As one noted, "We were really good." Another admitted, "We thought we were elite, we had information others did not have, we understood the EKG, we could do things."[58]

This sense of professional distance from other nurses came from the almost natural inclination of nurses in hospitals to imitate the institutional social hierarchy. Among nursing care workers, educational level and social class served as stratifying criteria, as evidenced by the lower status accorded aides and practical nurses by graduate nurses.[59] Because of what they knew and what they could do, nurses in the special care units gained a status different from that of nurses who remained on the wards.[60]

Although diagnosis and treatment were traditionally considered the realm of the physician, nurses in intensive care units proved that effective patient care could not be rendered unless they had the authority and expertise to use these skills.[61] One of the problems encountered by nurses and physicians was the length of time between discovery and diagnosis of patient problems and the initiation of treatment. Traditionally, nurses did not have the authority to independently initiate treatment of physically unstable patients without a physician's order. Thus unstable patients received treatment in a multiple-step process. Usually, the general-duty nurse called the nursing supervisor when patient problems arose. The supervisor came to see the patient, assessed the situation herself, and made the decision to call the physician.[62] The supervisor also called the physician, thereby excluding the staff nurse from the decision-making process. In this way, nursing supervisors acted as gatekeepers. They screened out unnecessary calls to physicians at night, especially from students and less skilled nurses, and protected staff nurses by assuming legal responsibility for order changes. However, this process lengthened the time between identification of a patient problem and a response.

Both physicians and nurses realized the risk the prolonged

decision-making process posed to physically unstable patients. After intensive care units formed, this process gradually changed. Through informal negotiations with physicians, nurses in the intensive care unit gained the authority to assess the patient's condition and call physicians themselves, thereby cutting out several steps of the process. "We were really good nurses," one nurse remarked. "We could decide [when] to call the doctor. . . . Doctors knew we knew what we were doing."[63] These negotiations accomplished several goals: patients received more intense observation in the physician's absence, physicians gained a greater sense of security for themselves and a greater margin of safety for their patients, and nurses gained greater authority for decision-making.

As did many other physicians, Dr. Lawrence Meltzer understood the importance of negotiated patient care responsibilities. After several months of operating a coronary care unit (CCU) at Presbyterian Hospital in Philadelphia, he contacted Dorothy Mereness, then dean of nursing at the University of Pennsylvania, and asked her to recommend someone qualified both to teach nurses about coronary care and to take charge of the unit. Dean Mereness suggested Rose Pinneo, who began working at Presbyterian Hospital in July 1963 as the associate director of the cardiac care unit. Together, Lawrence Meltzer, Rose Pinneo, and the other nurses worked together as a team, teaching, conducting research, and providing patient care. Rose Pinneo remembered, "We really worked together as a doctor-nurse team. Dr. Meltzer had confidence that nurses could do things, we could monitor, we could identify arrhythmias. The success was partially due to his philosophy."[64] In fact, as Meltzer and Pinneo note in the preface to the first edition of the classic *Intensive Coronary Care*, coronary care is "not an advanced system of medical practice based on electronics," but an advanced system of nursing care. This system relied on the authority derived from the negotiations between nurses and physicians to provide better care to their critically ill patients.[65]

The Patients

As part of the division of labor, patients in hospitals are able, at various skill levels, to protect themselves using information, personal contacts, and previous experience. As patients become sicker and more physically unstable, however, they are less able to use these skills or to participate in the work of getting well. Critically ill patients in particular are less able to manage their illness trajectory.[66] Doctors and nurses take on the tasks of illness management for the patient in the intensive care unit: these functions are then transferred back and forth from patient to caregiver, depending on the patient's level of illness. The presence of a cadre of skilled nurses and close working relationships between physicians and nurses facilitate this transfer.

The transfer process was particularly important during the twenty years following World War II as disease trajectories changed and medical advances were rapidly implemented. Until these decades, many diseases and chronic illnesses were treated by palliative, standard measures requiring concentrated nursing labor, rather than by quick diagnosis and decision-making. Typhoid fever patients, for example, required constant bathing and feeding. Nurses treated congestive heart failure patients by constantly rotating tourniquets among various limbs.

During the 1940s and 1950s, doctors prescribed newly available and more complex medications and performed complicated invasive techniques. Patients lived longer and suffered more complications and chronic illness. Those undergoing the treatments and experiencing the complications required nursing care beyond the functional procedures taught during training. Similarly, in order for the treatments to be as safe and effective as possible, physicians themselves had to learn about patient responses to treatments and had to rely on "expert" nurses, usually those found in the intensive care units, to monitor patients in the physicians' absence. For example, in the 1950s and 1960s, new sulfhydryl or ethacrynic acid diuretics were introduced for the treatment of congestive heart failure. Although the diuretics worked well, they sometimes induced rapid, severe hypovolemia and electrolyte disturbances. Physicians relied on nurses to observe closely patients' urine output, weight, and laboratory studies to anticipate problems. To keep patients safe, nurses had to make quick and accurate assessments, report the findings to a physician, and quickly respond to physician orders.

Word of the success of patient care negotiations, the resultant shared responsibility, and the effect on patient safety through improved mortality was at first passed on through stories related by individual nurses and physicians, similar to the way folktales were spread. Eventually, in the 1980s, research studies pointed to the success of collaborative ties between nurses and physicians (as measured by patient mortality or other parameters of patient outcomes) in numerous settings such as hospitals and primary care settings and in the treatment of certain conditions such as chronic pain and AIDS.[67] The importance of shared responsibility for patient safety and outcomes has been most clearly documented by researchers in intensive care units.[68]

Conclusion

The history of the invention of the new nurse and of the negotiation of work boundaries between nurses and physicians reveals strong and continued dependency on circumstance, local initiatives, and individual personalities. Thus the boundaries of work changed in an ad hoc manner, making it difficult for both professions to legislate or codify clear-cut work organization. Although states now attempt to specify the professional activities of doctors and nurses through professional practice acts, the boundaries of the actual day-to-day tasks of caring for patients remain flexible.

How work roles are negotiated is also quite dependent upon the participating parties and the situation. Power, gender, class, and race, among many other factors, influence the process and outcomes of the negotiations. Similarly, in emergency situations negotiations concerning actions may be more flexible, with nurses gaining more authority and responsibility by nature of their proximity to and knowledge of the patient.

The negotiations between doctors and nurses in the early intensive care units represented a break from many traditions. Although negotiations on the general floors also changed, they did so in a slower, almost reluctant manner, held hostage in part by the effects of educational socialization, economic forces, and control issues. A continued monopoly on decision-making by physicians in intensive care units would have been out of step with the realities of patient care and potentially dangerous to patients. Patients, nurses, and physicians themselves realized the potential for danger and the potential benefits to be realized by this new model of care. Although grouping sick patients with a reasonable quantity of expert nurses was not a novel approach, the additional authority

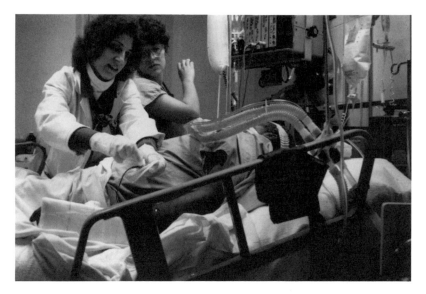

Figure 11. Nurses monitoring a critically ill patient, Hospital of the University of Pennsylvania, circa 1980. Courtesy of the School of Nursing, University of Pennsylvania, Philadelphia, Pa.

and decision-making capabilities negotiated by nurses represented a radical care alternative.

The concept that alternatives to traditional work boundaries and relationships existed and were exercised added to the power of the intensive care unit. The range of who could make choices and how choices were made created a pooling effect of knowledge, experience, and skill. All parties benefited within the intensive care zone. While at home, in the operating room, or elsewhere in the hospital, physicians gained a greater sense of security about the care of their physically unstable patients. In order for this security to be realized, physicians and nurses had to renegotiate the boundaries of patient care work. In the process, physicians ceded certain of their traditional tasks to nurses.

Nurses negotiated from a level of power. They had gradually gained expertise and experience in caring for unstable patients and had become indispensable in an environment of complex patient care and new technologies and treatments. Although nurses in general aimed for better patient care as an outcome of their negotiations, they also enjoyed the power and authority that came with the new work territory, oftentimes at the expense of those nurses who remained on the general units.

Chapter 5
From General-Duty Nurse to Specialist

When critical care nurses appeared in America's hospitals in the late 1950s, they quickly became major players in the rapidly expanding specialization of nursing practice. Many nurses began to redefine the boundaries of their own personal practices and, in the process, developed new forms of specialty practice in the field. Soon after launching the initial experiments in intensive care, proponents of these practice reforms began looking for both informal and formal means to differentiate their practice from general nursing practice and existing specialties.

In particular, hospital nurses sought to contest the then-prevailing idea that any nurse should be both able and willing to care for any patient, at any time, anywhere in the hospital. Hospital administrators and directors of nursing strongly preferred flexibility among their nursing staff; they wanted to be able to move a nurse from one area of the hospital to another as needs for staff dictated. The universal norm for hospitals was to have generalists who could and would practice anywhere. This traditional expectation was supported by educators and administrators. In the hospital, where unrelenting economic and clinical pressures to deliver continuous nursing care to a wide variety of patients called for an interchangeable and flexible workforce, the "nurse of all trades," whether still a student or a general-duty graduate nurse, was expected to perform competently wherever and whenever called upon.

As noted earlier, however, some leaders in hospitals were beginning to believe that nurses must have specialized expertise to assure the safety of hospital patients, especially those with life-threatening illnesses. The precedent of operating room and recovery room nurses combined with pervasive specialism inherent in midcentury medical practice began to spur changes in the traditional expectations of nurses. Moreover, hospital leaders saw that the increased costs associated with a more differentiated, specialized nurse workforce might be passed on to third-party payers through insurance.

A New Specialty Organization

The founding and subsequent development of the American Association of Critical-Care Nursing (AACN) provides an excellent case example for studying the late-twentieth-century nursing specialization movement. Before the AACN was organized in 1969, knowledge and oversight of the care of the critically ill and the management of intensive care units depended on local, scattered, and disparate groups of innovative nurses and physicians who communicated with each other in an occasional and haphazard fashion. Once the AACN was created, its leaders quickly moved to fill the information and organization gaps that coincided with fast-moving, widespread, and radical changes in nursing and medical care of the critically ill.

Historian Sydney Halpern argues, "[Professions] come into being through the efforts of practitioners who build new types of careers amid changing social and economic circumstances."[1] This observation works equally well for specialists branching off from a larger specialty organization. Certainly the intensive care units of the 1950s and 1960s provided a fertile environment in which to nurture a new specialty in nursing. Constant social interaction and communication among nurses and physicians, and in some cases hospital administrators, who shared a common interest in care of the critically ill helped to form mutual agreements on new patterns of work. A special location in the hospital with which practitioners could identify, the intensive care unit, helped nurses conceive of themselves as new and different professionals. Special skills and knowledge acquired through training and frequent practice led to new thinking about the nurses' scope of practice. Their expanded responsibilities created a new definition of what would become "normal" and expected expertise on the part of certain nurses. And, of course, implementing therapies and procedures that saved lives added to the nurses' mystique and helped to verify their distinctiveness in the eyes of others.

Many nurses volunteered to practice in the new intensive care units. The AACN leaders we interviewed from the early units often spoke of seeking out the "best" nurses in the hospital and encouraging them to ask for assignment to the new intensive care unit. In other cases, however, nurses were assigned to intensive care in a fairly traditional manner by their superiors, that is, they were involuntarily rotated to the intensive care unit from other parts of the hospital.[2] Such nurses often actively or passively resisted the responsibility and extra work involved in learning and executing new skills.

The administrators who insisted that any nurse could practice in the new units were simply continuing to act on their preference for highly mobile, general-duty hospital nurses. They thought of critical care nursing as just one more general-duty skill. The oscillating "busyness" of the intensive care unit and the higher nurse-to-patient ratio tempted administrators to pull nurses out of intensive care when it was less busy. Relying on generalist or rotating staff, however, meant unpredictable skill and knowledge levels among the nurses who were actually assigned to care for unstable, complex patients. Placing variously prepared nurses into intensive care at busy times became less common as the dangers of doing so became more evident. Gradually, if erratically, philosophical assumptions about the best ways to staff different types of patient care units began to change.

Skilled nursing was, after all, the key component of intensive care, making it nonsensical to try to staff the units with less-skilled nurses who either did not want or could not handle the added responsibility. Apparent relatively quickly was the necessity of establishing a stable nursing staff—nurses who worked in intensive care all the time. These nurses, who identified themselves as intensive or coronary care nurses, constituted the first cohort of critical care specialists.

Favorable Conditions for Specialization

Intensive and coronary care nurses were by no means the only nurses naming themselves as special or different in the late 1960s and early 1970s. Nurses who specialized in the care of people with kidney disease (nephrology nurses) organized a specialty group in 1969. Nurses working with cancer patients organized their own first Cancer Nursing Conference in 1973. By 1975, with the intent of educating and locating other nurses working in their field, cancer nurses founded the Oncology Nurses Society.

Nursing's boom in specialization was due partly to the fact that money was available to support differentiation of hospital nursing practice. Medical historian George Rosen, one of the first to draw the connection between medical specialization and affluence, pointed out the key aspects of the connection, arguing that "differentiation among healers is dependent on economic conditions," and "the accumulation of an economic surplus [is needed] to support them while they are carrying on their professional activities."[3] U.S. affluence in the 1950s and 1960s, manifested in the Johnson Administration's Great Society funding for health projects and spreading health insurance benefits, created the economic base to support nursing differentiation. New types of nursing work, new technology, higher public expectations of the health care system, funds to support higher education, and professional ambition spurred nurses to select specific arenas of nursing expertise in which to develop their individual careers.[4]

One forerunner of nursing differentiation, specialized education for psychiatric nursing built on a base of general nursing, emerged after World War II. Nurses learned their craft in psychiatric hospitals dating from the beginning of the twentieth century. The major change after World War II was that advanced education in psychiatric and mental health concepts was built on a general nursing base and intended to prepare nurses for therapeutic rather than only custodial work with patients. The expansion of the scope of required nursing knowledge and expertise in mental health nursing was spurred on by public concern about widespread mental illness discovered in young men serving in the military. Moreover, the public was scandalized by stories of the poor care received by patients in the nation's many mental health institutions; the deplorable conditions depicted in the popular post–World War II movie *The Snake Pit* epitomized the public concern. The National Mental Health Act of 1946 appropriated money for nurses who chose to obtain graduate degrees in psychiatric–mental health nursing. Nurses took advantage of the public funds available for higher education, and nurse specialists in psychiatric–mental health nursing began to develop a wide array of specialized practices. Thus, through a combination of public concern and willingness to commit resources, psychiatric nurses differentiated their practice from general nursing as their colleagues in public health nursing and industrial nursing had done earlier in the century.

Like the critical care nurses, however, the majority of early nurses who decided to specialize learned their skills on the job, not in school. Most pioneer critical care nurses, nephrology nurses, and oncology nurses have similar recollections. Usually nurses collaborated informally with physicians to establish the medical and nursing boundaries of patient care responsibility in the specialty. Nurses sharing specialty interests often first met one another at medical meetings where they went to learn more about clinical innovations and often also gained support and encouragement from nursing and medical colleagues around the country for their changing practices at home. Several of the nursing specialty groups founded in the 1960s and 1970s trace their origins to the gathering together of interested nurses at meetings of their medical specialist colleagues.

Pioneer specialist nurses trained their helpers and successors via the apprentice method; later, they devised educational programs based in hospitals or with medical specialty organizations. Quite often, specific training sessions at these locations were sponsored by equipment or drug manufacturers. Some educational programs were underwritten by federal or private-foundation funds; some were very informal demonstrations over a patient's bed. In the beginning, the mantle of competence assumed by the nurse specialist was based on accomplishment witnessed and attested to by physicians and other nurses rather than on any particular educational or professional credentials.

As early as 1952, the National League for Nursing, the professional organization that sets and oversees standards for nursing education, recommended that specialty preparation should be at the master's level.[5] However, in spite of the NLN's position on the matter, for the next fifteen years few master's programs in nursing actually offered clinically grounded content or experience. Most focused instead on training for teaching and administration. The exceptions were the few clinical specialist programs in psychiatric–

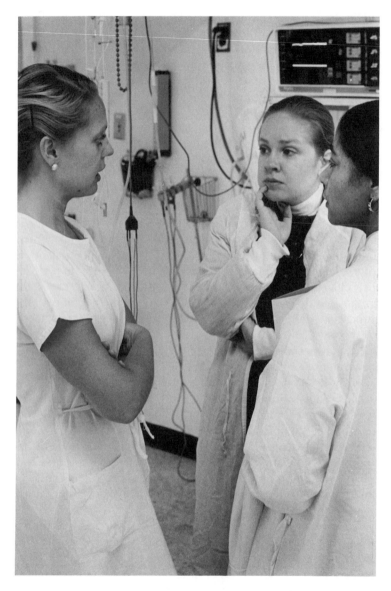

Figure 12. A concerned trio of nurses, Hospital of the University of Penn-sylvania, circa 1980. Courtesy of the School of Nursing, University of Pennsylvania, Philadelphia, Pa.

mental health nursing. After 1963, when a chain of political decisions led to legislation mandating funding via the Division of Nursing in the United States Public Health Service for training clinical nursing specialists, master's level nursing education finally was reformed in the nation's university-based nursing schools.[6]

The intent of the federal funding was to ensure that better educated and more experienced nurses would deliver direct patient care, rather than to prepare nurses only for administration and teaching as had been the pattern for a generation. Master's-prepared clinical nurse specialists appeared first in psychiatric–mental health, maternal–child health, cardiopulmonary, and oncology nursing. In the mid-1970s, critical care and nurse practitioner programs of study began to be offered at the master's level. Placing these programs at the graduate level meant that new specialists' training could be built on the natural and social science base and general nursing education obtained in baccalaureate study. By the late 1980s, slightly more than 80 percent of all nurse practitioners were being prepared in graduate programs.[7]

The idea of a nurse specialist as a direct caregiver caught on only after some initial delay during which these newly minted expert nurses figured out what their jobs were. Even after the federal subsidy for general nursing education began to be cut back in the late 1970s, graduations from specialty master's programs continued to grow. In 1969, seventy universities across the nation offered master's programs in nursing; ten years later, the NLN reported 125 programs.[8] One estimate asserts that, just in the three years between 1977 and 1980, the number of clinical nurse specialists jumped from 9,928 to 17,626 and the number of nurse practitioners and midwives grew from 3,296 to 5,500.[9] This was happening within a context of rapid growth in master's and doctoral preparation for nurses; by 1986, more than 100,000 nurses held master's or doctoral degrees; by 1992, the figure reached 150,728.[10]

Spreading Specialism

Professional reaction to the nurse specialist phenomenon was mixed; it was similar in many ways to attitudes toward medical specialization earlier in the twentieth century. Many nurses and nurse educators were skeptical of early nurse specialists. They thought nurse specialists were becoming too medical and charged that they were abandoning the broad, caring role of nursing. The relationship between the generalist nurse and the specialist provided the basis for plenty of debate among educators and the nursing leadership.

Predecessors of this debate were the critics of medical specialists, who also charged that, by narrowing their field of practice, physicians abandoned their obligation to know general medicine.[11] The rapid growth in numbers of medical specialists after World War II (medical specialists outnumbered generalists by four to one in 1975) lent some credence to criticisms of specialization. Many critics now argue that the ratio of physician specialists to generalists should be reversed. At issue was, and is, the proper mix of generalists and specialists to respond appropriately to the medical and overall health care needs of the society.

The specialization of medicine influenced the course of the expanding specialization of nursing in several ways. First, clinical nurse specialists and nurse practitioners moved into the gaps in patient care left when physicians specialized and moved away from generalized practice. Primary care nurse practitioners providing ambulatory health care are the best example of this. Other nurses took up new clinical work opportunities associated with new therapeutic modalities such as life support for premature infants or organ transplantation. Nephrology nursing, for instance, grew out of new treatments such as chronic renal dialysis and renal transplantation for formerly fatal kidney failure. These treatments created a whole new class of partially cured patients with complex, chronic needs for nursing care.

Nurse practitioners attracted public support when they proved able and willing to provide general care for a public lacking primary care services when physicians began to specialize and fewer of them chose general practice. Nurse midwives gained favor with the public by emphasizing intimate, low-technology, and personalized care during pregnancy and parturition. Midwifery priorities were in sharp contrast to hospital-based obstetric practices, which came to be seen by some of the public as increasingly impersonal and oriented toward high technology.

The nursing specialties that substituted nurse services for specialized physician services, such as nurse midwives and nurse anesthetists, sorted out their practice opportunities through a series of protracted struggles with physicians. In spite of the conflict the positions of both midwives and nurse anesthetists grew stronger after 1970 because they could offer good clinical care acceptable to patients at a reasonable fee in an increasingly cost-conscious health care system.[12] An experimental approach seemed to pervade the newer nursing specialties in the 1960s and 1970s. Especially in these early years, new nurse specialists and nurse practitioners tended to experiment with new roles and to make adaptations in both their practice and their education based on their experiences and the environments in which they found themselves.[13] There was no overarching plan; rather than following any set design, they tested ideas for organizing and delivering care. In general, self-declared nurse specialists moved into areas where they found least resistance from physicians or other nurses, such as the new health maintainance organizations (HMOs), kidney dialysis units, community mental health centers, neighborhood health clinics for the poor, and, of course, intensive care units. Late in this period (1980), gerontologic nurse practitioners and specialists began to appear in response to a prevailing sense of crisis related to care of the elderly.[14]

Setting Standards

In the 1970s specialty organizations took on the responsibility of setting practice standards and developing certification examinations for their respective areas of practice. The American College of Nurse-Midwives established exams in 1971, the American Association of Critical-Care Nurses developed exams and began to certify practitioners in 1976, and the National Board of Pediatric Nurse Practitioners and Associates followed suit in 1977. The precedent for much of this standard setting in specialty nursing was established by the American Association of Nurse Anesthetists, which began certifying nurse anesthetists in 1946.

Once specialized practice is recognized, a debate very quickly develops about who will authorize or guarantee competent advanced practice within the new specialty framework. Should such guarantees be the obligation of the larger professional organization (in nursing, the ANA)? Should it be the specialty organization, or perhaps the state licensing authority? Since credentialing is tied to the individual professional's ability to practice and to receive payment for services, control of credentialing is vitally important to the safety of prospective patients as well as to the practitioners' careers. The question of who has authority to credential the newer specialty practices has been hotly debated for the last twenty-five years. At this writing, the larger, established specialty organizations seem to be most effective at standard setting and testing for their constituents while the ANA maintains an active, national credentialing program. Many states, however, exercise their prerogative to oversee professional practice and place a variety of restrictions or controls on specialty practice in nursing through their medical and nursing regulatory authorities.

Developing the AACN

Unlike the national nursing organizations, ANA and the NLN, which are responsible respectively for protecting the interests of all professional nurses and developing and maintaining standards in nursing education, specialty organizations focus on clinical issues in their selected areas of nursing practice. A close look at the first two decades of the American Association of Critical-Care Nurses gives a good indication of which priorities were thought most important by early leaders.

In fact, the AACN decision to form a new organization separate from the ANA stemmed from vital and polarizing differences in mission. Nurses leading the AACN were most worried about clinical care issues in their own particular specialty, while the ANA leaders concentrated on global issues relevant to all nurses in the profession. Both the ANA and the AACN had to deal with the threatened splintering effect of specialization on the national body of nursing.

Defining the Specialty

As reported in Chapter 1, nurses interested in critical care, with impetus from Nashville nurse Norma Shephard and physician Fred Owenby, organized themselves at a cardiology meeting in 1968 in Nashville, Tennessee, as the American Association of Cardiovascular Nurses (AACN). The first AACN board members laid out the goals of the infant association in the fall of 1969 when they met at Baptist Hospital in Nashville. They declared that they were going to develop educational standards and techniques, cooperate with other organizations, publish periodicals, establish a central bureau of information, and disseminate knowledge about critical care through educational programs.

For two years, the founders referred to themselves as cardiovascular nurses—a term derived from their status as experts in care of patients with cardiovascular problems, especially coronary artery disease. The logo of the new AACN was a picture of a heart and its vessels framed against the earth. In a short time, however, the implications of confining themselves to the term "cardiovascular" began to be questioned by nurses who cared for critically ill patients with problems not related to the heart. By 1972, the group was ready to change its name to the American Association of Critical-Care Nurses; the hyphen made it possible to retain the original acronym.

In retrospect, two aspects of the budding culture of the AACN seem to be reflected in the decision to change the name of the organization. One aspect of the organization's culture is inclusiveness; the AACN from then on showed an organizational preference for a broad and inclusive, rather than exclusive, membership. Building on that first decision to include nurses who did all kinds of intensive care, the leaders of the organization consistently chose to grow larger rather than to become an elite specialty via narrow selectivity. Between 1971 and 1972, membership more than tripled, rising to 9,200 members.

The new name also signaled the AACN leaders' intention to differentiate their field from general or other specialty nursing practice on the basis of shared interest in a nursing care concept, that is, critical illness, instead of in a disease or organ system, the traditional models of medical differentiation. The internal debate over the new organization's name mostly revolved around the issue of scope of practice. Some nurses felt that full capability and expertise in cardiovascular nursing was all that could be expected of them. They thought that if the new organization took on a broader vision—critical care—the quality of education and standards for cardiovascular nursing would be compromised. They were not alone in their concerns.

When the name change from "cardiovascular" to "critical care" nurses was suggested to medical colleagues, who had provided much support to the early nurse leaders, the physicians were appalled. For physicians, concepts related to specific organs or to localized pathology seemed the only comprehensible, intellectual basis for specialization.[15] The decision-making AACN nurses, however, believed that confining themselves intellectually and professionally to organ systems or specific diseases would limit attainment of their broader clinical and educational goals. In this crucial instance, they chose to ignore the advice of their physician colleagues.

In 1969, Donna Zschoche and Lillian Brown outlined intensive care nurses' specific learning needs in the *American Journal of Nursing*, the widely read official nursing journal. Intensive care nurses, they asserted, used physiological and technological knowledge to anticipate critically ill patients' reactions, modified treatment plans based on interpretation of physiological data, and were capable of exchanging work and information with physicians. The authors believed that nurses would be able to meet these requirements via basic nursing preparation and experience, supplemented by special continuing education.[16] This special continuing education, which was not really available anywhere else, became the focus and mission of the early AACN.

In spite of its small size and lack of staff, the AACN cranked out ten newsletters to its membership in 1971. The newsletters spread word of conferences and courses, urged members to recruit other nurses, sought involvement of members in the AACN, and shared clinical information. Essay topics ranged from how to recognize patient anxiety or aberrant electric impulses in the heart to the industrial nurse's responsibility for the employee with a myocardial infarction.[17] In January 1972, after more than a year of negotiation, AACN's new official publication, *Heart and Lung: The Journal of Critical Care*, was published for the first time.[18]

The nagging problem of how specialty organizations like the AACN could work out their relationship to the ANA was still unresolved. In 1973, the AACN leadership invited other national nursing organizations to a meeting called the "National Nurses Congress," held at President Richard Nixon's "Western White House" in San Clemente, California. The National Nurses Congress was intended to be a forum for communication, mutual support, and cooperation among nursing specialty groups and a means for them to hold a conversation with the ANA. According to AACN's executive director, Donna Zschoche, the purpose was to "join to accomplish for nursing those objectives impossible to do singularly."[19]

The contemporary National Federation for Specialty Nursing Organizations (NFSNO), a loosely structured coalition of large and small nursing organizations, is an outgrowth of the 1973 San Clemente meeting. The NFSNO meets twice a year; its main function is to link together diverse specialties so they can communicate with each other and with the professional organization, the ANA. The AACN has been, from the beginning, the largest of the represented specialty organizations. The American Association of Operating Room Nurses, the American Association of Nurse Anesthetists, and the Nurses Association of the American College of Obstetricians and Gynecologists are the only other groups of comparable size.

The NFSNO has, at times, been seen as a threat by the ANA because it is a functioning coalition of the representatives of the very large number of nurses who belong to the various specialty organizations. Often, nurses hold memberships in both their specialty organization and the ANA. Questions of authority over credentialing, claims that specialty organizations draw members away from the ANA and craft unified political positions for nursing, and a long list of other concerns complicate the relationship between the specialty groups and the ANA. Over the years, however, most issues eventually have been resolved through discussion and compromise.

Education for Critical Care

Early AACN committees focused almost exclusively on education; they formulated plans for a curriculum for teaching critical care, developed an achievement examination, and started work on an innovative national teaching institute scheduled to take place in 1974. In just four years after the first AACN board meeting in Nashville, the association had addressed all the founders' goals. Astonishingly, it had also grown from the original 140 nurses to over 16,000 members.

Beginning with the first National Teaching Institute, held in New Orleans in 1974, which attracted 2,757 registrants, the AACN embarked on several years of intensive educational effort.[20] The

National Teaching Institutes, familiarly referred to as the "NTI," have been fabulously successful, drawing huge crowds of nurses to educational and motivational sessions and providing substantial revenue for the AACN each year. For the first decade or so these were overseen by Wanda Salas, an AACN staff member with a genius for organizing. Salas set a high standard for the NTI, making it the "must" meeting to attend. The NTI remains an important socializing event for nurses entering the specialty and a highly visible platform for association members. Local and national conferences, publications, standard setting, and certification became the main work of the constantly growing organization.

AACN members wrote a core curriculum for critical care that outlined the knowledge essential for practicing critical care nursing. Section headings listed cardiovascular, respiratory, neurological, renal, endocrine, and psychosocial content, accompanied by case studies to demonstrate the "total system approach." The curriculum was advertised in the AACN journals *Heart and Lung* and *Focus*, and disseminated through local chapters. The first thousand copies of the curriculum guide sold out in just a few months and the AACN rushed to prepare more. The enthusiasm of nurses for AACN's first National Teaching Institute and core curriculum as well as for the organization itself was clear evidence that AACN leaders were hitting the right notes with hospital nurses.

In 1981, the board of AACN took on the controversial issue of the basic educational standard for entry into professional nursing practice. For some fifteen years or longer U.S. nurses had been debating the merits of requiring the baccalaureate degree (B.S.N.) as the prerequisite for professional licensure and practice. According to Marguerite R. Kinney, AACN president in 1980, the proposal to raise the standard of entry was a particularly troublesome issue for the organization. AACN surveyed a sample of its members; a bare majority agreed to the baccalaureate standard. Arguing that the AACN must ensure individual professional accountability, thorough knowledge of life sciences and social sciences, appreciation of humanistic concerns, and "appreciation of the collaborative role of all members of the health care team," the AACN board resolved in its statement on entry into practice that the "minimal preparation for entry into professional nursing should be the baccalaureate degree in nursing."[21] Sympathetically and in detail, the resolution acknowledged the problems the position created for the nurse who was not baccalaureate prepared. The board's position was completely consistent with the association's habitual stance favoring higher educational standards for nurses.

A Growing and Confident Association

The AACN position paper on entry into practice was just one of nearly three dozen such papers put out by the association on various topics, ranging from scope of practice and relationships with physicians to education and ethics. As its membership grew, AACN became ever more conscious of its capability to do more than just offer its members specialized education. Its first position paper, issued in 1976, staked out the practice territory of the critical care nurse. Titled "Prevention of Fragmentation of Patient Care: The Coordinative Role of the Critical-Care Nurse," the paper asserted that the "registered, professional critical-care nurse is responsible and accountable for the coordination and implementation of physician-ordered care, nursing, and care delivered by allied health personnel in the critical care unit, and that the critical care nurse should be the recognized coordinator of caregiving resources in order to promote excellence in the care of the critically ill." The AACN was responding to the confusion and competition among multiple workers in intensive care units, especially the various therapists and technicians. Someone had to be in charge of the unit, and the AACN insisted that the "someone" was going to be the nurse.

The ongoing series of position papers constituted AACN's reconstruction of authority and working relationships within the critical care unit. "Prevention of Fragmentation" was followed by a 1981 statement outlining the principles of critical care nursing practice, a 1983 position on the use of technical personnel in critical care settings, a 1984 definition of critical care nursing, and 1986 statements on the scope of critical care nursing practice and role expectations for the critical care manager. In 1987, AACN put out a detailed description of the critical care clinical specialist, defining the expectations of the master's-prepared expert practitioner/teacher. In 1990, the role of the critical care nurse as patient advocate—described as personally and professionally risky—was outlined and encouraged.

Throughout the 1980s, the AACN position papers mark a trail

of developing confidence and clarity about critical care nurses and their relationship to other health care workers and to patients and their families. In 1983, the organization tacitly recognized the significance of its growing external influence by codifying its process for addressing practice, political, and professional issues. All such issues brought to the AACN for action were screened by the president who delegated responsibility for determining relevance and priority.[22] The resulting position papers could then be used by nurses or nurse educators around the country to substantiate their own efforts to improve care or training. No other organization effectively competed with the AACN for the role of standard setter for critical care. By 1990, AACN membership had grown to 65,000; the association's impact was powerful indeed.

The AACN has, over time, almost always worked closely with physician groups in an effort to avoid confrontation and emphasize collaboration. In addition to the important founding roles of physician colleagues, an early example of this is the production of a statement on collaborative practice that the AACN issued in conjunction with the Society of Critical Care Medicine in 1982. The two groups called for physician and nurse directors in critical care units to operate on an equal decision-making level to ensure that optimum patient care was achieved. On the other hand, the AACN leaders were quick to criticize the American Medical Association when it tried to limit the functions of nurses in hospitals and curtail federal funding for nurse education.[23]

Perhaps the most crucial accomplishment of the AACN was to define, demonstrate, and codify the component parts of nursing expertise, thus making measurable standards possible for its own special area. Its curriculum and credentialing work, combined with usually judicious statements of position on issues, established something of a model for late-twentieth-century specialty organizations in nursing.

During the 1980s research into fundamental issues affecting care of the critically ill became part of the AACN agenda. An example of this was the "AACN Demonstration Project," which set out to investigate the cost effectiveness of critical care nursing. Using data derived from patients and physicians as well as nurses in selected study units, the project's comparisons indicated that adhering to high quality standards reduced expected patient mortality and did not raise costs.[24] This particular research direction

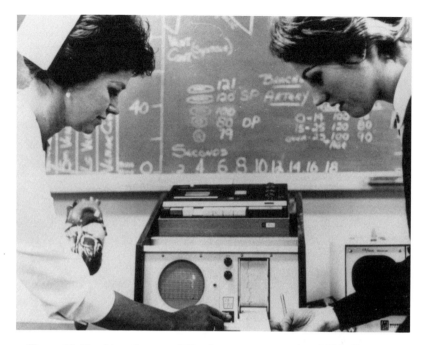

Figure 13. Teaching the new skills of coronary care, circa 1960. Courtesy of the U.S. Public Health Service Historical Collection, *HSMHA World.*

was influenced by increasing public recognition that the critical care system had to take into account not only patients' desires and needs, but also their ability to benefit from care. Better information about nurses' and physicians' effectiveness, they hoped, would encourage better use of resources. By 1990, the AACN made research an explicit value, focusing on expanding the scientific base for critical care nursing practice as well as improving general understanding of critical care practice on patient outcomes.

Establishing Critical Care Nursing

The most nuanced contemporary definition of expertise in nursing can be found in the work of Professor Patricia Benner, who writes that the precise hallmark of the expert lies in his or her proven ability to read patients' patterns of need for nursing care, immedi-

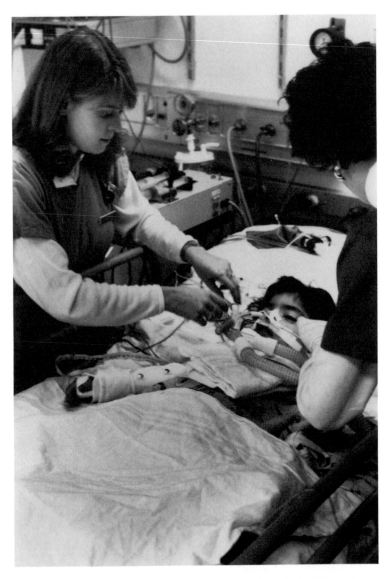

Figure 14. Teaching critical care nursing, Hospital of the University of Pennsylvania, circa 1980. Courtesy of the School of Nursing, University of Pennsylvania, Philadelphia, Pa.

ately grasp the care requirements of each person, and then take action appropriately.[25] The thirty-year specialization movement in critical care nursing, led by a wide variety of nurses and coordinated by the AACN, markedly increased the probability that any critically ill patient in today's hospitals will receive at least some of his or her care from a nurse expert in critical care instead of having to rely on a less expert generalist nurse. Although concerns about cost and overtreatment persist, the validity and desire for expert nursing is attested to by the public and by a steady stream of studies confirming the life-preserving impact of critical care nurses.

Chapter 6
At Century's End

Our current concept of critical care nursing is based on the remedies formulated to repair the inadequate hospital nursing and medical care systems of the 1950s. New therapeutics, changing popular ideas of appropriate amenities in care, growing expectations of survival in the face of illness, willingness to alter traditional medical and nursing practices, and, above all, the public's willingness to spend money on medical care all nourished the evolution of critical care. Nearly fifty years of experience with critical care innovation leaves us with new understandings; some are encouraging while others demand sober reflection.

Critical care does work to save lives, maintain bodily functions, and implement complex therapies. As a treatment modality— a total technology—it has lived up to its promise that intense monitoring and correct interventions during periods of physiological instability will help many people get through otherwise deadly medical crises. Maintaining heart action and blood circulation, respiration, kidney function, and balanced body chemicals and gases, while keeping the skin whole and the brain protected, through many kinds of medical crises is now seen as almost commonplace. Television shows such as *ER* and *Chicago Hope*, for instance, might make us think that critical care is inevitably successful.[1]

We know, however, that surviving a critical illness is neither commonplace nor inevitable. For a person to survive profound losses of physiological function requires an elaborate assembly of people, machines, and medicines all working and being used in timely coordination. The zone of safety for the patient begins with access to critical care precisely when he or she needs it. Access means being

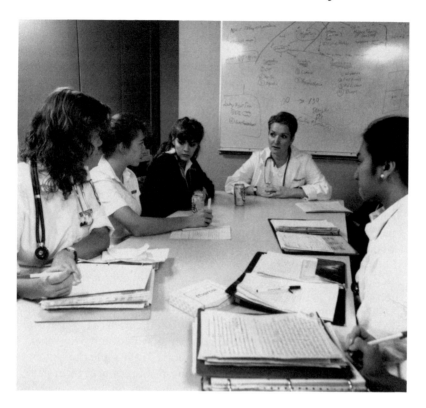

Figure 15. Critical Care Unit, Children's Hospital, Philadelphia, circa 1980. Courtesy of the School of Nursing, University of Pennsylvania, Philadelphia, Pa.

close enough to a critical care center that is competent to successfully treat the illness if treatment is possible and desirable. Access to critical care may also mean having the knowledge, will, and the financial resources to obtain such care when it is needed.

Two generations of physicians and nurses worked to master the many intricacies essential to make the critical care technology succeed. Even where critical care is unquestionably desirable, however, it is not always up to standard or, in some cases, care standards are still underdeveloped.[2] Spreading the word on new modes of treatment and improved technology or drugs takes time and money. Changing the beliefs and habits of practitioners, however expert they may be, calls for research, documentation, and dissemination of the desired change.

Our years of experience with critical care may also have erased the memory of formerly commonplace sudden hospital death from shock, cardiac arrthymia, kidney failure, or respiratory arrest. But the impotence of health professionals confronted with such problems and stripped of their technology is clear at the scene of any remote automobile accident or on visiting a hospital in a less developed country. Understanding the interdependence of expert nurses and their technology is crucial to thinking about critical care. Survival of life-threatening illness or accident is never commonplace; however, for the first time in history, it is now a choice to be made, at least for some.

For critical care, which can keep people alive, forces the question of when and when not to employ the full gamut of life support—when to use critical care for its original purpose. People suffering from terminal illnesses so severe that death is expected in weeks or months may not wish to subject themselves to intensive care in order to stay alive. Instead, they may wish for pain relief, comfort measures, and emotional support. At the same time, questions arise as to whether the life-saving resources of critical care units should be expended on people who can obtain no benefit from treatment.

More fundamentally, critical care accentuates and enables a tendency long noted in American health care ideology—the supremacy of curing disease and prolonging life over all other considerations.[3] The invention of and massive investment in critical care and critical care nursing was, one could argue, simply a manifestation of the power of that ideology. Even now, critical care remains the most expensive and fastest growing type of care offered in hospitals. Care of patients in intensive care units has, for some years, consumed up to 20 percent of the nation's hospital budget or almost 1 percent of the gross national product. More importantly, this resource is consumed by only a small fraction of the population.[4] Americans place a high value on health and would prefer not to confront death and disability. It should be no surprise that nurses and physicians in critical care would seek to do everything possible for their patients.[5] Given that death can often be forestalled (although at exceptionally high cost), the question remains whether we can find a more nuanced and complex way of viewing critical care.

For several years—beginning about 1992—the AACN sought to encourage nurses toward a broader concept of critical care by promulgating the idea of a "patient-driven system" of care.[6] The fact that AACN leaders thought the system needed to be made to be "patient-driven," of course, suggests they recognized that the experience of receiving critical care had become frightening, overly mechanistic, and not friendly to patients and families. The crux of the patient-driven concept was that patient and family needs should be paramount—that nurses and physicians would see the "health care experience through the eyes of the patient and his family."[7] The AACN leadership urged greater emphasis on the principles of coordination of care, patient and family education about clinical status, physical comfort, pain control, emotional support, involvement of family and friends, and problems of transition to other settings.

In particular, the expert nurse is expected to place his or her patient in a technical and physiological context, interpreting the meaning of the patient's illness and treatment to the patient, and helping the patient and his or her family understand what is happening and about to happen. Of course, the expert nurse must, at the same time, be completely knowledgeable about the sciences and adept in the skills of critical care. Moreover, the patient-driven approach calls for collaboration between nursing, medicine, and all other involved disciplines to share in the concept and reorient care priorities according to its principles.

In a logical extension of the idea of a certified expert critical care nurse, leaders and educators in the field turned to the critical care nurse practitioner (CCNP) in the 1990s. The CCNP is a master's prepared clinical expert in the care of people who are physiologically unstable and technology dependent. Critical care nurse practitioners function as case managers who work in close collaboration with the patient's physician. Systematically recognizing the overlap of skills and knowledge between specialized nurses and physicians suggests that more CCNPs will improve prospects for making critical care available in the coming years.[8]

The issue of how to apportion critical care in ways that are appropriate and sensitive to the many aspects of individual welfare will not be easily resolved, however. The actions of the AACN, the interest and research support of major foundations and professional groups, and the broad public interest in end-of-life questions may well yield better answers in the future. At the least, these fundamental questions are today being raised and debated in multiple forums.

Critical Care Nursing Now

Over the last two decades, critical care nurses and other nurse specialists created and then began to sort themselves into categories coined "intensivists" and "consulting nurse specialists" by health policy scholar Linda Aiken in her analysis of hospital nursing.[9] As described earlier, different groups of specialized nurses identified themselves and developed their scope of practice in similar ways. Specialization in nursing is still fluid and highly dynamic; it reflects the close and responsive links between nursing practice and the kind of care the public seeks during illness.

Intensivists or critical care nurses are trying to articulate a clearer picture of their practice as it is driven by patient needs. Nurses argue that there is "no more basic [patient] need than the need for competent nurses."[10] The return of the AACN to its earlier emphasis on competence can be understood as a response to recent efforts to reduce costs in delivering hospital services by cutting back on the number and qualifications of nursing personnel. Specialist nurses strongly believe that safe care depends on experts working directly with patients. They resist the idea of lesser trained, less expensive personnel taking responsibility for complex patient care tasks.

Major questions remain regarding work boundaries and negotiations between nurses and physicians. How will the current insurance restrictions on the decision-making of physicians influence relationships between nurses and physicians? How will physicians' increasing sense of loss of control over patient decisions and their own practice influence their negotiations with nurses? Physicians still hold a great deal of power in the health care arena; nurses continue to rely on personal initiative and the individual willingness and goodwill of physicians to participate in shared patient care decision-making. As more medical territory falls in the realm of "shared" jurisdiction, it will be harder for physicians to justify their fading monopoly over patient care decisions. Reallocating authority for critical care could well increase tensions between the two professions.

Reducing the number of nurses in hospitals and relocating more seriously ill patients outside of hospitals is forcing the AACN and other specialty organizations to think through once again the standards and location of their practice. As more people obtain complex care in their homes and families assume new burdens, some critical care nurses may well relocate their practice to their patients' homes.

Wherever care is to be given, the relentless demands of physiologically unstable, critically ill patients for expert and sensitive care poses four perennial questions for nursing:

- What should every professional nurse be able to know and do for every patient—the well or convalescing, the very young or very old, the critically and dangerously ill?
- What should select specialist nurses be expected to know and do for each of these categories of patients?
- Where and how should the generalist nurse and the specialist nurse learn their respective roles; that is, what should be taught to all undergraduate nurses and what should be reserved for graduate education?
- How many generalist nurses and how many specialist nurses do we need?

Two generations of nurses have sought answers to these questions for the critically ill and for all those who require nursing care. The task is not complete. In fact, these issues will never be permanently resolved because our health care system continues to change in response to demographic shifts, the strength of the economy, new knowledge, new technology, and changing social preferences about the use of scarce resources.

Nursing the critically ill reflects our society's desire to sustain life whenever possible and to give hope and comfort to the sick and their families. The conundrum is that care of the sick is difficult, complicated, protracted, fraught with unintended consequences, and appallingly expensive. The history of care of the most seriously and critically ill must, by necessity, reflect all of these problems. But that history also gives testimony to the endurance and power of human ingenuity and caring.

Abbreviations

AACN	American Association of Critical-Care Nurses
CHH	Chestnut Hill Hospital, Chestnut Hill, Pa.
CHHSON	Chestnut Hill Hospital School of Nursing Collection, Center for the Study of the History of Nursing, School of Nursing, University of Pennsylvania, Philadelphia
CSHN	Center for the Study of the History of Nursing, School of Nursing, University of Pennsylvania, Philadelphia
HUP	Hospital of the University of Pennsylvania, Philadelphia
NL Coll	Nadine Landis Collection, Center for the Study of the History of Nursing, School of Nursing, University of Pennsylvania, Philadelphia
OPGE	Office of Post Graduate Education, HUP, Philadelphia

Notes

Chapter 1: Inventing Critical Care Nursing

1. In this book we will follow the lead of the 1983 NIH Consensus Conference on Critical Care Medicine (U.S. Department of Health and Human Services, National Institutes of Health, *Consensus Conference on Critical Care Medicine* [Washington, D.C.: GPO, 1983], 277) and not distinguish between the terms "intensive care units" and "critical care units." We will call all of the early units "critical care units" to consistently identify them. Most of the early units were not retrospectively regarded by their participants as critical care units because of the simplicity of the environment. Special care room, intensive room, and critical room were some of the frequently used names for the "first generation" of intensive care units.

We will also rely on the definition of critical care units presented by the Consensus Conference: a critical care unit is capable of "providing a high level of intensive therapy in terms of quality and immediacy . . . to patients who have sustained or are at risk of sustaining acutely life-threatening single or multiple organ system failure due to disease or injury" (p. 277). Although this definition may appear advanced for the circumstances of the 1950s, it is appropriate when judged by standards of intensity, quality, and immediacy appropriate to the 1950s. For example, a high level of intensive therapy in the 1950s may have included frequent blood pressure measurements by nurses, blood transfusions, or low nurse to patient ratios, rather than computer measurement of blood arterial gases or cardiac index.

We will also use the terms "physiologically unstable patient(s)" and "critically ill patient" interchangeably, as does the Consensus Conference report.

2. William U. McClenahan, *GP* (Philadelphia: Dorrance and Co., 1974), 114. In subsequent references, Hospital of the University of Pennsylvania, Philadelphia, will be referred to as HUP, and Chestnut Hill Hospital, Chestnut Hill, Pennsylvania, will be referred to as CHH.

3. American Hospital Association, "Annual Guide Issue," *Hospitals* 34 (1 August 1960): 394.

4. American Hospital Association, "Annual Guide Issue," *Hospitals* 40, part 2 (1 August 1966): 467. Cardiac care units were not yet factored out of the general intensive care unit total in 1966.

5. Louisa May Alcott, *Hospital Sketches* (Boston: James Redpath, 1863), 47.

6. Florence Nightingale, *Notes on Hospitals*, 3d ed. (New York: Longman, Green, Longman, Roberts, and Green, 1863), 89.

7. Quoted with permission from Jacqueline C. Zalumas, "Critically Ill and Intensively Monitored: Patient, Nurse, and Machine—The Evolution of Critical Care Nursing" (Ph.D. diss., Emory University, 1989), 105.

8. Robert R. Cadmus, "Special Care for the Critical Case," *Hospitals* 28 (September 1954): 65; idem, "Intensive Care Reaches Silver Anniversary," *Hospitals* 54 (16 January 1980): 98–102.

9. William J. Grace, "Determinants of Successful Cardiac Resuscitation," in *Proceedings of the Conference on Impact of Coronary Care Unit on Hospital, Medical Practice, and Community* (Arlington, Va.: National Center for Chronic Disease Control, 1966), 14.

10. Esther Lucile Brown, *Nursing for the Future: A Report Prepared for the National Nursing Council* (New York: Russell Sage Foundation, 1948), 12.

11. Some suggested that the number of active private-duty nurses fell by more than 40 percent during World War II. Mary M. Roberts, *American Nursing: History and Interpretation* (New York: Macmillan Co., 1954), 363.

12. Max S. Sadove, James Cross, Harry Higgins, and Manuel J. Segall, "The Recovery Room Expands Its Services," *Modern Hospital* 83 (November 1954): 65–70.

13. Julie Fairman, "When the Emergency Was Routine" (speech delivered at the American Association for the History of Nursing annual conference, Cincinnati, Ohio, 1988).

14. Vickie Wilson, "From Sentinels to Specialists," *American Journal of Nursing* 90 (3) (October 1990): 32–43. Aramine was a drug used at the time to elevate blood pressure; it was important to administer it at a controlled rate so that blood pressure would not rise precipitously or fall too low.

15. By the late 1920s, Dr. Walter Dandy's neurosurgical patients were cared for "around the clock" by special nurses in a small room next to his neurosurgical operating room at Johns Hopkins (A. McGehee Harvey, "Neurosurgical Genius: Walter Edward Dandy," *Hopkins Medicine* 135 [November 1974]: 364–65). Indeed, the idea had been around for a long time. After his death in 1916, University of Pennsylvania surgeon Dr. James William White left one-third of the residue of his estate for the maintenance of beds in a special hospital ward for the "care of patrons immediately after grave surgical operations" (Annette Matkowski, "James William White, M.D., Ph.D., LL.D.," in *Annual Report of the Harrison Department of Surgical Research and the Department of Surgery* [June 1971], 5).

16. For a comprehensive description of the response to the epidemic, see H. C. Lassen, "Preliminary Report on the 1952 Epidemic of Poliomyelitis in Copenhagen," *Lancet* 1 (1960): 37–40; Bjorn Ibsen, "The Anesthetists' Viewpoint on Treatment of Respiratory Complications in Poliomy-

elitis During the Epidemic in Copenhagen," *Proceedings of the Royal Society of Medicine* 47 (1954): 72–80.

17. U.S. Army Medical Department, *Surgery in World War II*, vol. 1, *Thoracic Surgery* (Washington, D.C.: Office of the Surgeon General, Department of the Army, 1963), 91–93, 202.

18. Rosalie Hammerschmidt Lanius, one of the American Association of Critical-Care Nurses (AACN) founding leadership group, interview with Joan Lynaugh, 15 May 1989, Atlanta, Ga.

19. Probably more units opened in 1953 or 1954. However, their accounts remain unpublished. Nathan M. Simon to J. Don Miller, letter (undated), Chestnut Hill Hospital (CHH); Lewis E. Weeks, *The Complete Gamut of Progressive Patient Care in a Community Hospital* (Battle Creek, Mich.: W. K. Kellogg Foundation, 1966), 16–17; Elizabeth A. Bell, "Special Nursing Unit Relieves the Strain," *Modern Hospital* 83 (November 1954): 74–75; Sadove et al., "Recovery Room," 65–70; Cadmus, "Special Care," 65–66. The Index Medicus included the intensive care unit as an independent heading in the 1955–1959 issue.

20. The units differed in several ways. For example, the University of North Carolina Hospital unit only admitted children. Most units usually contained medical and surgical adult patients.

21. See Esther Claussen, "Categorization of Patients According to Nursing Care Needs," *Military Medicine* 116 (March 1955): 214. Claussen discussed a category of patients that required intensive nursing care, but did not address the spatial arrangement of patients according to that classification. Progressive patient care is further discussed by Lewis E. Weeks and John R. Griffith, eds., *Progressive Patient Care: An Anthology* (Ann Arbor: University of Michigan, 1964); Weeks, *Complete Gamut*; Faye G. Abdellah and E. Josephine Strachan, "Progressive Patient Care," *American Journal of Nursing* 59 (May 1959): 649–55; Lewis Weeks, ed., *Faye Abdellah in First Person: An Oral History* (Chicago: American Hospital Association Research and Educational Trust, 1983); U.S. Public Health Service, Division of Hospital and Medical Facilities, *Elements of Progressive Patient Care: A Tentative Draft*, pub. no. 59-9467-A (Washington, D.C.: GPO, 1959).

22. Weeks, *Complete Gamut*, 25.

23. See, for example, the photographs in the following articles: Theodore Last, "Connecting on the Critically Ill," *Hospitals* 86 (June 1956): 69–71; Sadove et al., "Recovery Room," 65; J. Murray Beardsley and Florence Carvisiglia, "A Special Care Ward for Surgical Patients," *Nursing World* 131 (March 1957): 11; CHH archives, photo collection, Medical Library.

24. Norma Shephard and Penny Vaughan, founding leaders of the AACN, interview with Joan Lynaugh, 15 August 1989, Nashville, Tenn.

25. Zalumas, "Critically Ill," 95.

26. See Rosemary Stevens, *In Sickness and in Wealth: American Hospitals in the Twentieth Century* (New York: Basic Books, 1989), 254–55.

27. Raymond S. Duff and August B. Hollingshead, *Sickness and Society* (New York: Harper and Row, 1968), 123. For another, earlier example of this bargain, see Barbara Bates, *Bargaining for Life: A Social History of Tuberculosis, 1876–1938* (Philadelphia: University of Pennsylvania Press, 1992).

28. Quote is from William Mosenthal and David D. Boyd, "Special Unit Saves Lives, Nurses, Money," *Modern Hospital* 89 (December 1957): 83–86. The units described by Sadove et al. ("Recovery Room," 65–70), Jane Barton ("Round the Clock Nursing or Self-Service: Patient Care Is Based on the Medical Need," *Modern Hospital* 88 [June 1957]: 51–56), and Paul Safar, T. J. DeKornfeld, J. W. Pearson, and J. S. Redding ("The Intensive Care Unit," *Anesthesia* 16 [July 1961]: 275–84) did not admit terminally ill or unsalvageable patients.

29. The intensive care unit at HUP excluded ward patients until 1967. The university hospital studied by Duff and Hollingshead (*Sickness and Society*) also excluded ward patients.

30. Stevens, *In Sickness*, 253.

31. Shephard and Vaughan, interview, 15 August 1989.

32. Gloria Woolever Kundrat and Betty Lou Bridal, interview with Julie Fairman, 26 May 1989, Berwick, Pa.

33. Julie Fairman, "Watchful Vigilance: Nursing Care, Technology, and the Development of Intensive Care Units," *Nursing Research* 41 (January/February 1992): 56–60.

34. Rosemary Nocella, Polly Barrick, and Lucy Fort, "The Evolution of Critical Care Nursing" (unpublished manuscript at North Carolina Memorial Hospital, Chapel Hill).

35. See, for example, staffing cited by Harry T. Haver and Harry T. Haver Jr., "Subrecovery Unit Solved a Familiar Problem for This Hospital," *Hospitals* 31 (October 1957): 47–48; Beardsley and Carvisiglia, "A Special Care Ward," 11–13; Annual report of the Department of Nursing Service, HUP, 1959–1960, Nadine Landis Collection (hereafter cited as NL Coll) in the Center for the Study of the History of Nursing (hereafter cited as CSHN), School of Nursing, University of Pennsylvania, Philadelphia; Last, "Critically Ill," 69–71.

36. Lawrence Meltzer, Rose Pinneo, and J. Roderick Kitchell, *Intensive Coronary Care—A Manual for Nurses* (Philadelphia: CCU Fund, 1965), preface.

37. Quoted in Phillip Kalisch and Beatrice Kalisch, *The Advance of American Nursing*, 2d ed. (Boston and Toronto: Little, Brown and Co., 1986), 688.

38. Fairman, "Watchful Vigilance."

39. Joan Lynaugh, "Four Hundred Postcards," *Nursing Research* 39 (July/August 1990): 252–53.

40. Barbara Rollins, R.N., telephone communication with Joan Lynaugh, March 1990.

41. Lynaugh, "Four Hundred Postcards."

42. Lanius, interview, 15 May 1989.

43. Stevens, *In Sickness*, 296.

44. Christopher W. Bryan-Brown, M.D., and Kathleen Dracup, R.N., D.N.Sc., titled their November 1993 editorial in the *American Journal of Critical Care* "1993: A Precarious Year for Critical Care." In it they worry about high costs, overregulation, interprofessional competition between

medicine and nursing, and the difficulties of ethical decision-making. These themes persist through the 1990s.

Chapter 2: Hospitals in Transition

1. Rosemary Stevens, "A Poor Sort of Memory: Voluntary Hospital and Government before the Depression," *Milbank Memorial Fund Quarterly* 60 (1982): 557–58; idem, *In Sickness*, 40–46.
2. Stevens, "Poor Sort of Memory," 568.
3. Duff and Hollingshead, *Sickness and Society*, 36.
4. Ibid., 37.
5. Ibid., 35–43.
6. Minutes of the Medical Board, Hospital of the University of Pennsylvania (HUP), Philadelphia, 15 October 1951, Office of Medical Affairs, HUP.
7. Stevens, "Poor Sort of Memory," 557–58. Stevens documents nineteenth- and early-twentieth-century court cases granting tax exemptions and cross-subsidization to voluntary hospitals.
8. President's Commission on the Health Needs of the Nation, *Building America's Health*, vol. 3 (Washington, D.C.: GPO, 1953), 31.
9. Figures are from the Health Insurance Institute, *Source Book of Health Insurance Data, 1963* (New York: Health Insurance Institute, 1963), 11. Statistics from the U.S. Department of Health, Education, and Welfare, Public Health Service, *Medical Care Financing and Utilization: Source Book of Data through 1961*, Health Economics Series no. 1 (Washington, D.C.: GPO, 1962), 95–96, also demonstrate the rapid increase in the insured population.
10. Stevens, *In Sickness*, 259.
11. American Hospital Association, "Annual Guide Issue," *Hospitals* 44, part 2 (1 August 1970): 473.
12. American Medical Association, "General Report," in *Commission on the Cost of Medical Care* (Washington, D.C.: American Medical Association, 1964), 142, 146.
13. Herbert E. Klarman, *The Economics of Health* (New York: Columbia University Press, 1965), 39. The change in percentages may be due to inclusion of indigent aged patients covered by the Kerr-Mills legislation of 1960. Stevens, *In Sickness*, 273–75, discusses the expansion of services for the indigent elderly that occurred under Kerr-Mills. In the same source, Stevens also noted increasing hospital utilization by patients aged sixty-five and older, from 10 admissions per 1,000 persons (1921–1924) to 134 admissions (1955–1957), a 13-fold increase (p. 250, table 9.3).
14. American Medical Association, "General Report," 146, 165.
15. American Hospital Association, "Annual Guide Issue," *Hospitals* 26, part 2 (June 1952): 25.
16. Data were derived from various sources, such as the annual reports

of the Board of Managers, HUP, NL Coll., 1950–1960; Morbidity and Mortality Reports, 1950–1960, Department of Surgery, HUP, Office of Post Graduate Education (hereafter cited as OPGE), HUP, Philadelphia.

17. Data were derived from the minutes of the Medical Staff Committee, Board of Trustees, Chestnut Hill Hospital (CHH), Chestnut Hill, Pa., 1950–1960.

18. American Medical Association, "General Report," 160.

19. "Changes in Nursing from 1938 to 1953," *Nursing Research* 5 (October 1956): 85–86. Although this study covers the previous decade, it sets the trend for the 1950s.

20. Minutes of the Pharmacy Committee, Medical Board, HUP, 16 April 1956. The discussion of the committee centered around the use of newly available vials, which cost two hundred dollars more per year than tablets. The procedure is described in detail in the Philadelphia General Hospital School of Nursing's *Nursing Procedures* (Philadelphia: Philadelphia General Hospital, 1954), 71. The care of syringes is described briefly in "Care of Hypodermic Needles and Syringes," *American Journal of Nursing* 52 (March 1952): 297.

21. See J. Mostyn Davis, "Oxygen Therapy," *Modern Hospital* 79 (November 1952): 98–106.

22. A. N. Richards, "Production of Penicillin in the U.S. (1941–1946)," *Science* 201 (1 February 1964): 441–45.

23. Minutes of the Department of Surgery, HUP, 11 June 1956, OPGE.

24. Minutes of the Department of Surgery, HUP, 9 July 1951.

25. Minutes of the Medical Board, HUP, "Ad Hoc Report to Survey Spaces for Isolation Facilities," 20 October 1958.

26. Minutes of the Department of Surgery, HUP, 8 April 1957. Gloria Woolever Kundrat and Betty Lou Bridal also discussed the epidemic and the pain and discomfort of the staph lesions (interview with Julie Fairman, 26 May 1989, Berwick, Pa.).

27. Doris Carnevali and Nola Smith Sheldon, "How Early Ambulation Affects Nursing Service," *American Journal of Nursing* 52 (August 1952): 954–56.

28. Ibid., 955.

29. Bridal, interview, 26 May 1989.

30. University of California School of Nursing, *A Functional Analysis of Nursing Service* (San Francisco: University of California, 1950), 11–14.

31. Faye Abdellah, "Progressive Patient Care—A Challenge for Nursing," *Hospital Management* 6 (June 1960): 102–6, 135; Esther Claussen, "Categorization of Patients According to Nursing Care Needs," *Military Medicine* 116 (March 1955): 214.

32. Quote is from Faye G. Abdellah, "Progressive Patient Care," *American Journal of Nursing* 59 (May 1959): 649–55.

33. Stevens, *In Sickness*, 263.

34. Ibid.

35. Annual report of the Board of Managers, HUP, 1951–1952.

36. Stevens, "Poor Sort of Memory," 573.

37. Annual report of the Board of Managers, HUP, 1951–1952; minutes

of the General Staff Meeting of the Medical Board, HUP, 2 December 1959.

38. Minutes of the Medical Board, HUP, 15 December 1958, appendix D.

39. The characteristics of ward patients and the increased use of laboratory tests and X rays for them are discussed by Duff and Hollingshead, *Sickness and Society*, 348–50.

40. Annual reports of the Board of Managers, HUP, 1950–1960. The figure for days of care is an average over a ten-year span.

41. Minutes of the Medical Board, HUP, 25 November 1957.

42. Orville Bullitt to Donald Pillsbury, letter contained in minutes of the Medical Board, HUP, 20 January 1958, appendix F. The hospital's financial picture warranted concern. Although each recent financial year ended with a budget surplus, the actual amount was minuscule. For example, the year 1951 ended with a budget surplus of $497. Although the hospital ended the 1956 fiscal year with a $6,400 surplus, it was almost $5,000 lower than that of the year before (Annual reports of the Board of Managers, HUP, 1951–1957).

43. Minutes of the Medical Board, HUP, 15 December 1958.

44. In 1956, the Red Cross began to charge a two-dollar fee for blood. The medical board noted that, although this might cause bad public relations within the community, the fee should be charged to patients. The board suggested that the charge should be absorbed by the privately insured patient. The hospital would "absorb" the fee for those who could not pay (minutes of the Medical Board, HUP, 17 December 1956). Duff and Hollingshead describe similar practices (*Sickness and Society*, 40, 53).

45. Minutes of the Board of Trustees, CHH, 23 January 1951, CHH Library, Chestnut Hill, Pa.

46. Report of the Executive Director, in the minutes of the Medical Board, HUP, 18 October 1965. On the other hand, Rosemary Stevens noted that "relatively little care was actually given away" by voluntary hospitals, although she also argued that this quantity was difficult to estimate. When hospitals matched fees to expenses and showed a deficit, they conveniently ignored other sources of income (e.g., endowments, local tax breaks, and donations). See Stevens, *In Sickness*, 269.

47. Minutes of the Medical Board, HUP, 16 April 1962.

48. During the 1950s, "geographic full time" meant that a physician contracted with a hospital, in exchange for hospital admitting privileges, to practice solely at a particular institution. The physician collected fees directly from the patients, and paid expenses and office rent to the hospital. "Financial full time" meant that a physician received a salary and a certain percentage of his or her private practice contribution, the rest of which was turned over to the hospital (Jonathan Rhoads, interview with Julie Fairman, 2 April 1990, HUP). Rhoads also suggested that increased money from the National Institutes of Health for training grants contributed to the larger number of physicians on financial full time.

49. Report of the Professional Staff Committee, in the minutes of the Medical Board, HUP, 17 September 1956.

50. Physicians at HUP expressed numerous complaints about the waiting list for semiprivate rooms. (See report of the Department of Surgery, annual report of the Board of Managers, HUP, 1959–1960.) This scenario was influenced both by the increase in hospital utilization by insured patients and by the building program undertaken during this time, which necessitated closing of wards and older semiprivate floors during construction.

51. Minutes of the Board of Trustees, CHH, 27 November 1962. Duff and Hollingshead (*Sickness and Society*, 56–57) also discuss the reliance of private physicians in community hospitals upon interns and residents.

52. Edwin Albright, "Annual Report of the Director, 1961," Medical Department, CHH.

53. Report of the Training Committee, November 1955, Medical Staff Committee, CHH.

54. Minutes of the Medical Board, HUP, annual staff meeting, 5 April 1961.

55. Duff and Hollingshead, *Sickness and Society*, 40–45.

56. Ralph Perkins, telephone interview with Julie Fairman, 20 June 1990.

57. See John D. Thompson and Grace Goldin, *The Hospital: A Social and Architectural History* (New Haven, Conn.: Yale University Press, 1975), especially parts 2–4, for numerous examples of building and floor plans. It was also about this time that "ward" designation became "service" designation because the wards disappeared.

58. Clifford E. Clark, "Ranch-House Suburbia: Ideals and Realities," in *Recasting America: Culture and Politics in the Age of Cold War*, ed. Larry May (Chicago: University of Chicago Press, 1989), 179–90.

59. U.S. Congress, Senate Committee on Labor and Public Welfare, *Study of Health Facilities Construction Costs* (Washington, D.C.: GPO, 1972), 65. The Hospital Survey and Construction Act (Public Law 79-725), commonly known as the Hill-Burton Act, was signed into law by President Truman in 1946. The law provided direct financial support for community hospital development and attempted to set standards for construction. In Pennsylvania, the funds were earmarked for rural and psychiatric hospital development.

60. Quote is from "Advantages and Disadvantages of an All Private Room Hospital," Patient Care Committee, January 1961, HUP, NL Coll.

61. For a description of the process of conversion of English Nightingale wards to smaller units, see Thompson and Goldin, *The Hospital*, 231–32.

62. Robert Sommer, "Personal Space," *Canadian Architect* 5 (February 1960): 76–80; Hermann H. Field et al., eds., *Evaluation of Hospital Design: A Holistic Approach* (Boston: Tufts-New England Medical Center, 1971), refers to studies by J. T. Celatano, D. Amorelli, and G. Freeman (*Establishing a Habitability Index for Space Stations and Planetary Bases* [American Institute of Architects, 1963]) when planning room parameters for the Tufts-New England Medical Center.

63. U.S. Public Health Service, Federal Security Agency, *Blue Cross and Medical Service Plans,* by Louis S. Reed (Washington, D.C.: GPO, 1947), 33.

64. The proportion of ward contracts to the total ranged from 45 percent in the Michigan plan to 1 percent in the Philadelphia plan. The proportion depended upon the availability of semiprivate rooms and the number of beds each plan considered semiprivate. For example, southeastern states had few semiprivate beds but a large number of private and ward beds; therefore, ward contracts remained popular there until the mid-1950s. In the Pacific Northwest, rooms with three to four beds were considered wards, but in Philadelphia these rooms were considered semiprivate (U.S. Public Health Service, *Blue Cross,* 33–34).

65. At this hospital, the wards were fairly old, with a large indigent contingent that may have "shocked the sensibilities" of private patients (minutes of the Medical Board, HUP, 19 October 1953). Francis Wood, chief of medicine from 1947 to 1965, referred to the "hazards of the ward" (Francis C. Wood Collection, handwritten notes in folder marked "1953–1954," College of Physicians, Philadelphia).

66. For an overview of the urban exodus, see Jon C. Teaford, *The Twentieth-Century American City: Problem, Promise, and Reality* (Baltimore: Johns Hopkins University Press, 1986), 97–126. For the medical board's concern about suburbanization, see minutes of the Medical Board, HUP, 5 April 1961.

67. Joseph Lippincott to Dr. Thomas Fitz-Hugh Jr., letter, in minutes of the Medical Board, HUP, 9 October 1956, appendix B.

68. Dr. Thomas Fitz-Hugh Jr. to I. S. Ravdin, letter, in minutes of the Medical Board, HUP, 9 October 1956, appendix B.

69. Thompson and Goldin, *The Hospital,* 207.

70. Quote is from Mary Clymer's student log, 6 December 1887, Mary Clymer Collection, CSHN. Mary Clymer was a student at the Training School of HUP. She also is the nurse portrayed in the Thomas Eakin painting *The Agnew Clinic.*

71. McClenahan, *G.P.,* 113.

72. Quoted with permission from Zalumas, "Critically Ill and Intensively Monitored," 104.

73. National League for Nursing, "Consultation Visit, HUP, School of Nursing," 1959, NL Coll.

74. Maureen O'Hern, telephone interview with Julie Fairman, 7 March 1990.

75. O'Hern, interview, 7 March 1990.

76. Nurses' travel time was spent primarily on trips to rooms of patients who were critically ill. See Barton Burkhalter's response in National Academy of Engineering, *Costs of Health Care Facilities* (Washington, D.C.: National Academy of Science, 1968), 137–43.

77. Scottish Home and Health Department, *The Falkirk Ward,* vol. 4 (Edinburgh: Author, 1969).

78. Thompson and Goldin, *The Hospital,* 217.

79. The Nurseserver was a device in the wall of a patient's room that

was stocked with general supplies and that opened into both the corridor and the patient room; it was replenished daily by an aide or supply clerk (Gordon Frieson, "Integrated Communication through Construction," *Hospital Progress* 32 [August 1960]: 64–67). Examples of studies of communication systems include E. A. Jacobs, "Two Way Audible Communication," *Hospitals* 21 (October 1947): 44–45, and F. L. George and D. Popovitch, "What about a Voice Intercom System?" *Hospitals* 28 (February 1954): 80, both cited by Thompson and Goldin, *The Hospital*, 337. An example of the discussion of the number of oxygen outlets is found in J. D. Thompson, "How Many Oxygen Outlets?" *Modern Hospital* 92 (January 1959): 116–22.

Chapter 3: Nursing in Transition

1. Eleanor Lambertsen, interview with Joan Lynaugh, 13 December 1989, New York City.

2. The labels "staff nurse," "general-duty nurse," and "graduate nurse" are used interchangeably throughout contemporary literature of the time and consequently throughout this chapter.

3. Training nurses to care for physically stable patients was not wholly unreasonable. As Herman M. Somers and Anne R. Somers (*Doctors, Patients and Health Insurance* [Washington, D.C.: Brookings Institute, 1961], 65) and Rosemary Stevens (*In Sickness*) pointed out, more patients were admitted for hernia repairs, tonsillectomies, and hemorrhoid relief than for treatment of heart disease. The point is that patients with complicated and chronic illness, such as heart disease, represented a growing proportion of the hospital population and required far different nursing knowledge and skills than did patients needing hernia repairs.

4. Brown, *Nursing for the Future*. For an overview of nursing function studies, see "Twenty Studies of Nursing Functions," *American Journal of Nursing* 54 (November 1954): 1378–82; forty-three studies sponsored by the American Nurses Association and Foundation are summarized by Everett C. Hughes, Helen MacGill Hughes, and Irwin Deutscher, *Twenty Thousand Nurses Tell Their Story* (Philadelphia: J. B. Lippincott, 1958).

5. Marguerite Kinney, interview, May 1989, Atlanta, Ga.

6. Jean A. Curran and Helen L. Bunge, *Better Nursing: A Study of Nursing Care and Education in Washington* (Seattle: University of Washington Press, 1951), 133.

7. Elmina Mary Price, *Learning Needs of Registered Nurses* (New York: Teachers College Press, 1967), 38–41.

8. Everett C. Hughes noted that nurses' routines may be seen as a set of emotional and organizational checks and balances against the risks of their "trade," as protection against physicians' mistakes. See *Men and Their Work* (London: Free Press of Glencoe, 1958), 97. Zane Robinson Wolf also addressed nursing rituals in *Nurses' Work: The Sacred and the Profane* (Philadelphia: University of Pennsylvania Press, 1988).

9. Blood transfusion protocols at Hospital of the University of Pennsyl-

vania (HUP) in Philadelphia did not indicate that action should be taken if these symptoms occurred or address what the symptoms signaled (Nursing Technique Committee, "Blood Transfusion—Closed Method," 1954, School of Nursing, HUP, NL Coll). The procedure for blood transfusion at Philadelphia General Hospital School of Nursing (*Nursing Procedures,* 134) did not indicate symptoms to watch for, but noted, "Report untoward symptoms at once to the doctor so that the transfusion may be discontinued," without reference to the reason action should be taken.

10. Brown, *Nursing for the Future,* 10.

11. U.S. Department of Health, Education, and Welfare, Public Health Service, Division of Nursing Resources, *For Better Nursing in Michigan: A Survey of Needs and Resources* (Detroit: Cunningham Drug Co. Foundation, 1954), 34. Nationally, the change in the number of nurses in administrative and supervisory positions who had advanced skills cannot be determined. The number of nurses who graduated between 1950 and 1960 from baccalaureate programs that prepared for head nurse or other advanced positions actually declined 78 percent, due in part to termination of the Cadet Nurse Corps Program in 1949. However, the number of nurses who graduated from master's degree programs that prepared nurses for advanced positions increased 269 percent (only nonpublic health nurses included in the figures) (American Nurses Association, *Facts about Nursing: A Statistical Summary* [New York: American Nurses Association, 1961], 113–15; U.S. Public Health Service, Federal Security Agency, *The Cadet Nurse Corps, 1943–1948,* pub. no. 38 [Washington, D.C.: GPO, 1950]).

12. Hughes, Hughes, and Deutscher, *Twenty Thousand Nurses,* 135.

13. The study of small hospitals in Kansas noted the large array of tasks that nurses performed. See Governmental Research Center, University of Kansas, *The Study of Activities of Registered Professional Nurses in Small Kansas Hospitals* (Lawrence: University of Kansas, 1953), as cited by Hughes, Hughes, and Deutscher, *Twenty Thousand Nurses,* 127.

14. The paragraphs are from Claire Dennison, "Maintaining the Quality of Nursing Service in the Emergency Room," *American Journal of Nursing* 42 (July 1942): 774. Dennison is quoted extensively by others. Examples include Brown, *Nursing for the Future,* 80–81, and Mary M. Roberts, *American Nursing,* 335–36.

15. University of California School of Nursing, *Functional Analysis of Nursing Service,* 14.

16. Dennison, "Maintaining the Quality," 774. Eleanor Lambertsen echoed this theme in 1963 when she referred to nursing as "the waste basket of hospital services." See Eleanor Lambertsen, address given at the thirty-fourth Midwest Hospital Association Convention, 24 April 1963, Kansas City, Mo., cited by Rex W. Allen, "Designed for Nursing," *American Journal of Nursing* 64 (February 1964): 91.

17. American Hospital Association, "Annual Guide Issue," *Hospitals* 29, part 2 (August 1954): 102. Figures are for short-term, nonfederal, nonprofit housing.

18. Myrtle K. Aydelotte, *Survey of Hospital Nursing Services* (New York: National League for Nursing, 1968), 3.

19. Minutes of the Pharmacy Committee, HUP, 11 November 1959. The same issue plagued nurse supervisors at Chestnut Hill Hospital (CHH) in Chestnut Hill, Pa., where the director of nursing unsuccessfully attempted to spare them that time-consuming task (minutes of the Professional Staff Committee, Board of Trustees, CHH, 22 October 1963). The minutes offer no sign of resolution.

20. See, for example, Washington State Nurses' Association, *Nursing Functions Study: An Analysis of the Nursing Activities of a Medical Service* (Seattle, 1953), 93–94. This study of urban and rural hospitals was originally designed to develop an economical standard method to analyze nurses' work in any hospital. The data are based on more than nine hundred self-report diaries. Although this may somewhat limit the reliability of the study, other studies yielded similar results: New York University, *A Study of Nursing Functions in Twelve Hospitals in the State of New York* (New York: New York University, 1952); Donald Stewart and Christine E. Needham, *The General Duty Nurse* (Fayetteville: University of Arkansas, 1955), 69, 77; U.S. Public Health Service, Division of Nursing Resources, *How to Study Nursing Activities in a Patient Unit*, pub. no. 370 (Washington, D.C.: GPO, 1954), cited by Faye Abdellah, "Patient-Centered Approaches to Nursing Service," in *Patient-Centered Approaches to Nursing*, ed. Faye Abdellah et al. (New York: Macmillan Co., 1960), 42–45. Care must be taken with the figures of nursing function studies. For example, the category "activities with patients" includes "giving care" and "other direct activities."

21. Although function studies indicate trends, results should not be generalized because each study used different definitions of variables such as direct patient care. For example, the 1950 study by the University of California School of Nursing (*A Functional Analysis*) included time for paperwork in the direct care measurement; this study indicated that staff nurses gave more than 60 percent of their time to direct patient care. Study results, in general, were obtained in several different ways, including self-report (imagine a busy nurse attempting to complete an activities diary) and use of observers who may or may not have been nurses.

22. Robert P. Bullock, *What Do Nurses Think of Their Profession?* (Columbus: Ohio State University Research Foundation, 1954), 79.

23. Washington State Nurses' Association, *Nursing Functions Study*, 134.

24. Leonard Reissman and John H. Rohrer, *Change and Dilemma in the Nursing Profession* (New York: G. P. Putnam, 1957), 134.

25. Thomas R. Ford and Diane D. Stephenson, *Institutional Nurses: Roles, Relationships, and Attitudes in Three Alabama Hospitals* (University: University of Alabama Press, 1954), 348.

26. Team assignment or team nursing was not a new concept; it had been utilized since hospitals began employing different levels of nursing care workers. However, it was not until the late 1940s and early 1950s that the label "team nursing" became common. See Eleanor C. Lambertsen, *Nursing Team Organization and Functioning* (New York: Columbia University Teachers College, 1953).

27. Brown, *Nursing for the Future*, 82.

28. Jean Barrett, *Ward Management and Teaching* (New York: Appleton-Century-Crofts, 1954), 246–48; Dorothy Perkins Newcomb, *The Team Plan: A Manual for Nursing Service Administrators* (New York: G. P. Putnam, 1953), 33.

29. Kinney, interview, May 1989. Her recollections are from the mid to late 1950s. The team may have included one or two nurses (the team leader and a staff nurse). In general, the number of patients per nurse may be misleading. For example, the study by Ford and Stephenson, *Institutional Nurses*, indicated an average of five beds per graduate nurse, a seemingly low patient care load. However, the figure for graduate nurses included head nurses, supervisors, and the director of nursing.

30. Newcomb, *The Team Plan*, 20–21.

31. Mary Conneely Gorka, telephone interview, 7 March 1990.

32. Edna Reilly, interview with Julie Fairman, 28 March 1990, HUP.

33. Mimeographed sheets, Department of Nursing Service, HUP, "Nursing Service, 24-Hour Period for Two Weeks in May, 1958" (undated); the average patient census for May 1958 is from a hand-drawn graph, "Average Patient Census," Annual Report, 1964, Department of Nursing Service, HUP, CSHN. The figure of 84 students may be low. The 1958 National League for Nursing Progress Report for the School of Nursing, HUP, indicated an average of 154 students on clinical rotations per day.

34. Minutes of the Board of Trustees, CHH, 1949–1960; Pennsylvania State Board of Nurse Examiners reports, 1950–1960, CHH School of Nursing Collection (hereafter cited as CHHSON).

35. Gorka, interview, 7 March 1990. Some of the side effects of steroid drugs, such as prednisone, are mood swings and steroid-induced psychosis.

36. Medical Board, HUP, 17 June 1946 (abstracted in minutes of 19 April 1954).

37. For the recurring discussion of the relationship between students' clinical experiences and educational needs, see Isabel Maitland Stewart, *The Education of Nurses: Historical Foundations and Modern Trends* (New York: Macmillan Co., 1945), 213–16; Brown, *Nursing for the Future*, 138–73; Eli G. Ginzberg, *A Program for the Nursing Profession* (New York: Macmillan Co., 1948); Margaret Bridgman, *Collegiate Education for Nursing* (New York: Russell Sage Foundation, 1953), 36–69; Margaret West and Christy Hawkins, *Nursing Schools at the Mid-Century* (New York: National Committee for the Improvement of Nursing Services, 1950).

38. School of Nursing, HUP, "Factors Related to Nursing Student Experiences Which Have Influenced the Need for Increasing the Department of Nursing Staff," 3–4, 1971, NL Coll.

39. National League for Nursing, *Report on Hospital Schools of Nursing, 1957* (New York: NLN, 1959), 19.

40. One study indicated that students provided 43 percent of routine patient care, 50 percent of the bedmaking, 52 percent of the bathing, 33.3 percent of preparation for diagnostic procedures, 45 percent of the sterile treatments, and 35 percent of the intravenous medications. Washington State Nurses' Association, *Nursing Functions Study*, 32.

41. In 1957 at HUP, there may have been two ward instructors on evening shift and two on night shift to supervise and instruct approximately ninety students. The instructors were assisted by two evening and two night assistant instructors. These data are derived from a mimeographed sheet, untitled, detailing the average number of nurses, auxiliary workers, and students assigned for a twenty-four-hour period, during two-week surveys in May 1958, and from the School of Nursing Progress Report, part A, "Progress Made in Relation to Each Factor Indicated as Areas for Study and Improvement," 1957 (both documents, NL Coll).

42. Blanche Pfefferkorn and Charles A. Rovetts, *Administrative Cost Analysis for Nursing Service and Nursing Education* (New York: American Hospital Association and the National League for Nursing Education, 1940), 157; Lucile Petry Leone and Louis Block, *Cost Analysis for Schools of Nursing* (Washington, D.C.: U.S. Public Health Service, 1947) continued to use this figure in 1947.

43. Figures are derived from the annual service evaluations of the Department of Nursing Service, 1961–1964, HUP, NL Coll. These numbers are approximations because various sources present different counts of the number of graduates. The percentage of increase in nursing staff contributed by graduates is based upon the September figures of the number of nurses employed per month.

44. Figures are derived from the minutes of the Board of Trustees, CHH, "End of Year Report," 1947, 1953, 1955, 1960, and "Annual Report of CHH," 1964, 1965.

45. Report of the School of Nursing Committee, in minutes of the Board of Trustees, CHH, 22 February 1955 and 26 April 1955.

46. Minutes of the Board of Trustees, CHH, 25 March 1950. The value of student services does not take into account the expenses to the hospital of room and board. For example, in 1965 and 1966, the value of student services exceeded $100,000, but the hospital carried the schools at a deficit (State Board of Pennsylvania Nursing Survey for CHH, 1965, 1966, CHHSON). The hospital ended 1965 and 1966 with surpluses (approximately $24,000 and $76,000, respectively).

47. For the first four months of fiscal 1947, the hospital faced a budget deficit of $21,000. Similarly, the hospital faced a year-end budget deficit of $10,800 in 1948, but had surpluses of $8,700 in 1949, $17,000 in 1950, and $1,500 in 1951 (minutes of the Board of Trustees, CHH, "End of Year Report," 1948–1951).

48. Minutes of the Board of Trustees, CHH, 21 November 1944. The connection between the rise in nurses' salaries and in those of auxiliary workers continued through the 1950s. See, for example, minutes of the Board of Trustees, 22 October 1946: "Nurses' wages increased in line with those of other institutions, resulting in a $1,300 increase in the monthly payroll, plus about $300 additional for probable increases to other employees."

49. "Department Expenses by Comparison," CHH. The chart provides data from 1948 to 1952, and the trend is similar for each of the five years:

nursing expenses are lower than the state average, while both operation of plant, repairs, and upkeep and laboratory expenses are higher.

50. Minutes of the Finance Committee, Board of Trustees, CHH, 28 October 1947.

51. Minutes of the Board of Trustees, CHH, 11 October 1947.

52. Salary increases are noted in the minutes of 16 May 1944 and 22 October 1946 (Board of Trustees, CHH). A new Blue Cross contract was negotiated in November 1946. Salaries also included maintenance (e.g., room and board, laundry). An increased number of graduate nurses also meant an increase in maintenance fees. For example, the treasurer's report for January 1949 noted that the hospital would benefit from a gradual cut in expenses for graduate nurses because the student nurses would be back on the floor in February. He also suggested that the non-residential nurses (those living away from the hospital) be eliminated first because they received a thirty-dollar premium for living expenses not provided by the hospital. Also, these nurses could not easily be called back to work if they were needed.

53. In at least six instances between 1955 and 1965 professional nurse salary increases are followed closely (from two days to two months later) by room rate increases. The relationship is documented as early as 1950 (minutes of the Salary Committee, Board of Trustees, CHH, 19 December 1950). A letter from the president of the board of trustees to the medical staff documents the relationship: "Because of increased salaries to our nursing staff . . . we are forced to increase our room rates $2.00 per day for private and semiprivate patients" (28 February 1962, CHH).

54. Joseph C. Doane, "The Doane Report," 10 March 1948, CHH.

55. Ibid., unnumbered pages.

56. Ibid.

57. This figure probably represented turnover without replacement rather than discharged nurses; the nursing committee noted, "We are presently operating under a plan to not replace nurses who are leaving the hospital" (Minutes of the Executive Committee of the Board of Trustees, CHH, 22 March 1948).

58. Minutes of the Board of Trustees, CHH, 27 April 1948.

59. Minutes of the School of Nursing Committee, Board of Trustees, CHH, 29 October 1952.

60. Idem, 30 December 1952.

61. Pfefferkorn and Rovetts, *Administrative Cost Analysis*, 109; U.S. Department of Health, Education, and Welfare, Federal Security Agencies, Public Health Service, Division of Nursing Resources, *The Washington Nursing Survey*, appendix B (Washington, D.C.: GPO, 1950), no page number; National League for Nursing Education, Survey of the School of Nursing, 1950, HUP. The Pfefferkorn study of three hospitals noted that the norm for hours of care ranged from 2.3 hours for ward obstetric-newborn service to 6.5 hours for private obstetric (mothers) service. Medical and surgical services averaged 3.2 hours of care.

62. In 1948, preclinical courses for first-year students were moved to

Temple University (minutes of the Board of Trustees, CHH, 27 April 1948). This was a less expensive option than school-based instruction because two fewer instructors were needed and the students would be released two months earlier for general duty. The minutes also noted that other local schools, such as those affiliated with Germantown, Episcopal, Jewish, and Northeastern hospitals, were planning the same measures.

63. Minutes of the Executive Committee, Board of Trustees, CHH, 27 January 1953.

64. Minutes of the Finance Committee, Board of Trustees, CHH, 23 June 1953.

65. Ibid.

66. National League for Nursing, "1957 Accreditation Report for the School of Nursing, HUP," 26, NL Coll.

67. School of Nursing, School of Nursing Progress Report, part A, HUP, file marked "1957 resurvey," NL Coll.

68. The NLN offered one-day free consultation visits as part of the second phase of its "School Improvement Program" to schools not fully accredited during 1955–1957 accreditation visits. Mildred Schwier visited HUP's School of Nursing in February 1958. See National League for Nursing, "Report of the NLN Consultation Visit to HUP, School of Nursing," 11 February 1958, NL Coll.

69. National League for Nursing, "1958 Accreditation Report for the School of Nursing, HUP," NL Coll.

70. Although the hospital increased graduate staffing, it probably did not eliminate reliance on student staffing. One report discussed a new continuous care experience, noting that "it is advantageous to the student, but has caused some problems . . . the student actually assigned to the area is not there if the scheduled admission goes to another area. . . . Despite the fact that students are not used for service but are here for a learning experience, it does upset the Head Nurses' staffing pattern and plans" (monthly report of the Ravdin Building, Department of Nursing Service, 1–30 September 1963, 2, HUP, NL Coll).

71. Nursing Service Department, "Comparative Study of Nurse Staffing, 1930–1950" (undated), HUP, file marked "hospital statistics," NL Coll.

72. Values are estimated because data were derived from a hand-drawn graph. Annual report of the Department of Nursing Service, HUP, 1961–1962.

73. Logbook, Office of the Private-Duty Nurse Registrar, HUP, 23 October 1959, NL Coll.

74. Figure derived from various reports: Department of Nursing Service, 1960–1961; National League for Nursing resurvey of HUP School of Nursing, 1957, NL Coll; annual reports of the board of managers, HUP, 1950–1954.

75. Figures are from National League for Nursing, "Consultation Visit, HUP, School of Nursing," 1959, NL Coll. The 1958 figures for graduate nurses do not include the fifty head nurses on duty. The figures do include thirty-two nurses employed in the labor room, receiving ward, operating room, and outpatient department (and therefore may give an inflated

view of the numbers of general-duty nurses). The figures for numbers of private-duty nurses are derived from the annual reports of the board of managers, HUP, 1954–1960.

76. American Nurses Association, *Facts about Nursing: A Statistical Summary, 1956* (New York: American Nurses Association, 1957) 125. Private-duty registries received 31,000 more calls in 1955 than in 1950, but filled only 3,000 more in 1955 than in 1950. Figures are derived from table 1, which includes all types of registries. However, hospitals accounted for 98.6 percent of all calls received and 98.5 percent of all calls filled in 1955, so the figures are a fair approximation of the hospital scenario over the five years.

77. Last, "Concentrating on the Critically Ill," 69–71.

78. American Nurses Association, *Facts about Nursing: A Statistical Summary, 1956*, 86.

79. In 1960, 99 percent of all submitted private-duty requests were filled, but 70 percent of the requests on the 3–11 P.M. shift went unfilled. Annual report of the Department of Nursing Service, HUP, 1960–1961.

80. Minutes of the Department of Surgery, HUP, 19 June 1950.

81. Quoted from Duff and Hollingshead, *Sickness and Society*, 85.

82. Brooke Roberts, interview with Julie Fairman, 31 March 1990, HUP.

83. Logbook, Office of the Private-Duty Nurse Registrar, HUP, various entries; Bell, "Special Nursing Unit Relieves the Strain," 74, also notes that private-duty nurses at Albany Hospital routinely refused neurosurgical or thoracic surgical cases.

84. Logbook, Office of the Private-Duty Nurse Registrar, HUP, 30 November 1960.

85. Brown, *Nursing for the Future*, 13.

86. Roberta Spohn, "Some Facts about the Nursing 'Shortage,'" *American Journal of Nursing* 54 (July 1954): 865–66; Irene Butter, "The Supply of Nurses—Its Responsiveness to Economic Incentives," in *Hospital Nursing Shortage: Crisis or Illusion*, (Ann Arbor: University of Michigan Press, 1976), 42, 44. These figures are useful for indicating trends, not absolute descriptions. Figures are for all hospitals and all nurses.

87. U.S. Department of Health, Education, and Welfare, *Health Manpower Source Book*, sec. 2, rev. (Washington, D.C.: GPO, 1965), 89–90.

88. Ibid., 87; U.S. Department of Health, Education, and Welfare, Public Health Service, *Nursing Resources: A Progress Report of the Program of the Division of Nursing Resources*, prepared under the direction of Apollonia O. Adams, pub. no. 551 (Washington, D.C.: GPO, 1958), chart 1. This figure is for hospitals of all types. The figure for short-term general voluntary hospitals may be slightly lower because psychiatric hospitals were also hiring at rapid rates. See any of the annual guide issues of the American Hospital Association for related figures.

89. Annual reports of CHH and HUP, 1950–1961; Pennsylvania State Board of Nurse Examiners report, CHH, 1950–1960, CHHSON; annual report of the Department of Nursing Service, HUP, 1962; minutes of the General Staff Meeting, Medical Board, HUP, enclosure, 2 December 1959.

90. U.S. Department of Health, Education, and Welfare, Public Health

Service, *Nursing Resources*, chart 17. A 1955 study by the American Nurses Association (*Facts about Nursing 1955* [New York: American Nurses Association, 1956], 52) revealed a lower turnover of 42.2 percent for full-time graduate nurses. Eugene Levine ("Turnover among Nursing Personnel in General Hospitals," *Hospitals* 31 [1 September 1957]: 50–53, 138–40) suggested that the lower figure obtained by the ANA was caused by the large number of smaller hospitals (one hundred or less beds) with lower turnover rates that were included in the study.

91. Figures are derived from worksheets, 1954–1959, Personnel Department, CHH. The figures include both part-time (including part-time workers who did not work every pay period) and full-time nurses and auxiliary workers such as aides. Therefore, the number of nursing care personnel may be inflated, and the calculated turnover rate may be lower than actual. The actual turnover for auxiliary workers is unknown. Nationally, a 1955 rate of 70 percent for aides, orderlies, and attendants was presented by Levine ("Turnover," 51). Because of their lower educational level, they might be compared to personnel in the housekeeping or dietary department, which consistently reported the highest turnover of the hospital's eleven departments (between 100 and 150 percent turnover). However, the laundry, where one might speculate that personnel had the same educational level as auxiliary workers, reported turnover rates comparable to or only slightly higher than nursing.

92. Administrator's Report, in minutes of the Board of Trustees, CHH, 24 April 1956. The report does not indicate if both full- and part-time nurses are included in these figures, but we speculate that it includes both. Only an average of 133 nursing personnel were employed for that year, and an average of 28 nurses were scheduled per day in 1955.

93. Report marked "Hospital Nursing Survey," 1954, NL Coll.

94. Report of the Council of Teaching Hospitals, 26 February 1960, handwritten chart, NL Coll. HUP participated in the council.

95. Administrator's Report, minutes of the Board of Trustees, CHH, 24 April 1956.

96. Marvin Bressler and William Kephart, *Career Dynamics: A Survey of Selected Aspects of the Nursing Profession* (Harrisburg: Pennsylvania Nurses' Association, 1955), 52. The study indicated that 100 percent of nurses employed for less than three years had children. Forty percent of those with "high longevity" (employed for twelve to fifteen years) were childless.

97. Thomas McPartland, *Patterns of Career Dynamics in Nursing* (Kansas City, Mo.: Community Studies, unpublished), cited by Hughes, Hughes, and Deutscher, *Twenty Thousand Nurses*, 258–61.

98. Barbara Brush, "Percentage Distribution of R.N.s by Marital Status and Activity," unpublished chart, 1989.

99. Approximately 90 percent of the part-time nurses in one study were married, compared to 60 percent of all professional nurses. Eighty-five percent of part-time nurses had children. See Arthur Testoff, Eugene Levine, and Stanley E. Siegel, "The Part-Time Nurse," *American Journal of Nursing* (January 1964): 88–89.

100. Numerous studies and points of view emerged during this time

that attempted to explain the changes in women's role and status in the 1950s. Polar opinions about women's place in society and the labor force ranged from the neurotic female described by Ferdinand Lundberg and Marynia Farnham (*Modern Women: The Lost Sex* [New York: Harper and Brothers, 1947]) to Margaret Mead's awakening woman (*Male and Female* [New York: Morrow, 1947]). As William H. Chafe noted (*The American Woman: Her Changing Social, Economic and Political Roles, 1920–1970* [London and Oxford: Oxford University Press, 1972], 211–18), the debate occurred in a vacuum. Toward the middle and late 1950s, several studies emerged indicating that women derived satisfaction from their jobs through a sense of accomplishment, importance, and social relationships developed with other female coworkers. See, for example, Marion G. Sobol, "Commitment to Work," in *The Employed Mother in America*, ed. Ivan F. Ny and Lois W. Hoffman (Chicago: Rand McNally, 1963), 40–63; Robert Weiss and Nancy Samuelson, "Social Roles of American Women: Their Contribution to a Sense of Usefulness and Importance," *Journal of Marriage and the Family* 20 (November 1958): 358–66. Alice Kessler-Harris (*Out to Work: A History of Wage-Earning Women in the United States* [New York: Oxford University Press, 1982], 300–303) also discusses the trend in the 1950s of women working for "need," to help the family obtain a certain lifestyle and fight inflation.

101. Chafe, *American Woman*, 218. For a brief discussion of women in the labor force, see also Louis G. Galambos and Joseph Pratt, *The Rise of the Corporate Commonwealth: United States Business and Public Policy in the Twentieth Century* (New York: Basic Books, 1988), 180–81.

102. Bullock, *What Do Nurses Think*, 102.

103. Joan Wallach Scott, "The Problem of Invisibility," in *Retrieving Women's History—Changing Perceptions of the Role of Women in Politics and Society*, ed. S. J. Kleinberg (New York: Berg Publishers, 1988), 5–29. Scott briefly notes employers' "anticipation" of turnover in female labor forces and perception of women as "natural dependents" of men. She suggests that employers used these arguments to hire women at low wages. Her reference is to late nineteenth- and early twentieth-century women workers, but her point holds true from the 1940s to the present time. Kessler-Harris (*Out to Work*) suggests that women's cyclical work patterns related to marriage and childbirth began disappearing during the late 1940s and the 1950s due to the expanding economy and consumerism of the 1950s.

104. Annual report of the Board of Managers, HUP, 1965–1966, p. 3.

105. Ibid., 4.

106. Duff and Hollingshead, *Sickness and Society*, 383. Because positions were always readily available, nurses in this study did not report feeling anxious about changing jobs or leaving the workforce.

107. At HUP, almost all complaints about the shortage of nurses occurred from January to May. Complaints at CHH are somewhat more diffuse, but cluster around November through January (before the students completed their class work in February).

108. Mary Ross, "Private Life or Private Duty for the R.N.," *Survey* 60 (February 1921): 549–52, cited by Barbara Brush, "A Marriage of Conve-

nience: Group Nursing in United States Hospitals, 1918–1930," unpublished paper, 16 April 1991.

109. Hand-drawn graph dated 6 June 1962 in the annual report of the Department of Nursing Service, HUP, 1962.

110. Although figures for 1954 to 1957 do not exist, a symmetrical trend from 1958 to 1969 is evident, and conclusions may be drawn, carefully, for previous years (from hand-drawn graphs in the annual evaluation report of the Department of Nursing Service, HUP, 1962; "Number of Nurses, Inpatient Staffing, 1964–1969," HUP, NL Coll). The hospital census did not have much influence on the number of nurses employed. The census traditionally increased from February to March, when the number of nurses started to decline, creating a most critical time for patient care. The census then declined through August, following the decline of nurses. Census figures are available for 1958 to 1963. "Average Census," hand-drawn graph, in the annual report of the Department of Nursing Service, HUP, 1964.

111. Compare with note 110. Again, because the data include part-time nurses and auxiliary workers, the trend may be somewhat flattened. However, the same seasonal changes are seen at CHH, suggesting that a comparison is reasonable. Work sheets, Personnel Department, CHH, 1955–1959. Data from the Presbyterian Hospital in New York City, 1958–1959, also indicated similar seasonal patterns (Comptroller's Office, 4 February 1959, Presbyterian Hospital, New York, NL Coll).

112. "Analysis of Graduate Nurse Resignation, 1958," Nursing Service Department, HUP, NL Coll. See also Bell, "Special Nursing Unit Relieves the Strain," 74.

113. Hospital administrators (Ralph Perkins [20 June 1990] and Kenneth Wenrich [19 June 1990], telephone interviews with Julie Fairman) and a Department of Surgery chairman (Jonathan Rhoads, interview, 2 April 1990, HUP) suggested that for these reasons the hospital did not always hire as many nurses as it possibly could.

114. See Lambertsen's classic *Nursing Team Organization.*

115. Annual report of the Department of Nursing Service, HUP, 1963. This same theme of overlapping function in times of great demand (e.g., when faced with a large number of critically ill patients and few skilled staff) or according to the size of the hospital (occurring more frequently at small rather than large hospitals) is presented by Ford and Stephenson, *Institutional Nurses,* 37–45; Washington State Nurses' Association, *Nursing Functions Study,* 95–98.

116. Morris Wolf, "Practical Nurses—Letters to the Editor," *American Journal of Nursing* 52 (March 1952): 26.

117. HUP did not hire practical nurses until 1958 (annual report of the Department of Nursing Service, HUP, 1962). However, competition and resentment between registered nurses and practical nurses appeared to be prevalent in Pennsylvania. See Otto Pollak, Charles F. Westoff, and Marvin Bressler, *Pennsylvania Pilot Study of Nursing Functions* (Harrisburg: Pennsylvania State Nurses' Association, 1953), 10.

Both CHH and HUP tended to hire nurses' aides and ward helpers

rather than practical nurses. CHH relied heavily on Gray Ladies (female volunteers) and Red Cross aides, who were trained to take vital signs, do bed baths, and perform other routine functions, and who contributed from four thousand (1964) to ten thousand (1962) hours of volunteer work per year. Data are from annual reports of the Board of Trustees, CHH, 1960–1965; "[CHH]: Your General Hospital," *Chestnut Hill Local,* 9 May 1963, Chestnut Hill, Pa.
118. Letters are from *American Journal of Nursing* 52 (April 1952): 394 and 52 (June 1952): 664.
119. William H. Stewart, "The Surgeon General Looks at Nursing," *American Journal of Nursing* 67 (January 1967): 65.

Chapter 4: Negotiating New Roles

1. Gender, class, and economic issues surrounding nursing are major themes of two seminal analyses: Susan Reverby, *Ordered to Care: The Dilemma of American Nursing, 1850–1945* (Cambridge: Cambridge University Press, 1987), and Barbara Melosh, *"The Physician's Hand": Work Culture and Conflict in American Nursing* (Philadelphia: Temple University Press, 1982).
2. Charles Rosenberg, *The Care of Strangers: The Rise of America's Hospital System* (New York: Basic Books, 1987).
3. Ibid.
4. Barbara Melosh, "More Than 'The Physician's Hand': Skill and Authority in Twentieth-Century Nursing," in *Women and Health in America,* ed. Judith Walzer Leavitt (Madison: University of Wisconsin Press, 1984), 482–96. See also Robert Brannon, *Intensifying Care: The Hospital Industry, Professionalization, and the Reorganization of the Nursing Labor Process* (Amityville, N.Y.: Baywood Publishing Co., 1944), chap. 3.
5. Joan Lynaugh, "Narrow Passageways: Nurses and Physicians in Conflict and Concert Since 1875," in *The Physician as Captain of the Ship: A Critical Reappraisal,* ed. Nancy King, Larry Churchill, and Alan Cross (Boston: D. Reidel, 1988), 32. Lynaugh also notes how some nursing leaders saw the movement of nursing education into universities as a way of escaping physician control of training schools.
6. Ibid.
7. "Three Meetings and Their Messages," *Charities* 11 (25) (week ending 19 December 1903): 580.
8. Reverby speaks to the importance of the socialization of nurses as part of the patient therapy in *Ordered to Care,* 39–57. See also Hughes, Hughes, and Deutscher, *Twenty Thousand Nurses,* and Rose Laub Coser, *Life on the Ward* (East Lansing: Michigan State University Press, 1962). The socialization of physicians during their medical training is also documented by Rose L. Coser et al., *Boys in White: Student Cultures in Medical Schools* (Chicago: University of Chicago Press, 1961).
9. The expected behaviors of nurses toward physicians is found in Coser, *Life on the Ward,* 140–45, and in interviews with Kundrat and Bridal, 26 May 1989.

10. Interns and residents claimed they were too busy with an increased number of patients to remember to rewrite orders (e.g., restarting antibiotics or sedatives after three days, or new orders after surgery). Instead, they asked the medical board to have the nurses remind them when orders were needed (minutes of the Professional Staff Committee, Medical Board, Hospital of the University of Pennsylvania (HUP), Philadelphia, 18 February 1957).

11. Minutes of the Committee on Staph Infections, Medical Board, HUP, 17 February 1958.

12. Minutes of the Infection Control Committee, Medical Staff, CHH; 3 September 1958; memorandum by J. Don Miller to the Executive Committee of the Medical Staff, 18 April 1967, CHH.

13. Leonard Stein, "The Doctor-Nurse Game," *Archives of General Psychiatry* 16 (June 1967): 699–703. Stein later updated his observations: Leonard Stein, David Watts, and Timothy Howell, "The Doctor-Nurse Game Revisited," *New England Journal of Medicine* 322 (22 February 1990): 546–49.

14. Charles Bosk, *Forgive and Remember: Managing Medical Failure* (Chicago: University of Chicago Press, 1979), 61–63. See also Renee Fox, "Training for Uncertainty," in *The Student-Physician: Introductory Studies in the Sociology of Medical Education*, ed. Robert Merton, George Reader, and Patricia Kendall (Cambridge: Harvard University Press, 1957), 207–41.

15. Cheryl Larson, telephone interview with Julie Fairman, 7 September 1989.

16. Anselm Strauss et al., *Social Organization of Medical Work* (Chicago: University of Chicago Press, 1985), 274.

17. Strauss et al., *Social Organization*, 267. Strauss discusses negotiative work and how negotiations might entail a great number of sequences and tasks.

18. The need for nurses to prove their competency is noted by Claire M. Fagin, "Collaboration Between Nurses and Physicians: No Longer a Choice," *Academic Medicine* 67 (May 1992): 295–303, and by Patricia Prescott and Sally Bowen, "Physician-Nurse Relationships," *Annals of Internal Medicine* 103 (1) (July 1985): 127–33.

19. Anselm Strauss et al., "The Hospital and Its Negotiated Order," in *Profession of Medicine: A Study of the Sociology of Applied Knowledge*, ed. Eliot Friedson (New York: Atherton Press, 1970), 147–69.

20. American Association of Critical-Care Nurses, Kansas City chapter, interview with Hugh Day, 1987, *Kansas City Media Award Interviews* (unedited videotape).

21. Ibid.

22. J. Don Miller, "The Critical Care Unit in a 134-Bed Hospital," *Hospitals* 30 (16 October 1956): 46–47, 96.

23. J. Don Miller, interview with Julie Fairman, 26 March 1990, Roxborough, Pa.; Laura Mae Beery, interview with Julie Fairman, 22 January 1991, Chestnut Hill, Pa.

24. Miller, interview, 26 March 1990; J. P. Smith, memoranda on group private-duty nursing in intensive care units, 7 April 1961, CHH archives.

25. Miller, interview, 26 March 1990; Beery, interview, 22 January 1991.

26. Associated Hospital Services administered or brokered the local Blue Cross-Blue Shield plan, more commonly known as "Intercounty."

27. Miller, interview, 26 March 1990; J. Don Miller to E. A. Van Steenwyck, letter, 26 April 1954, CHH archives, file marked "intensive care."

28. Miller to Van Steenwyck, 26 April 1954.

29. Marian Bankert, *Watchful Care: A History of America's Nurse Anesthetists* (New York: Continuum, 1989).

30. Linda Aiken and David Mechanic address the danger of diverging interests in "A Cooperative Agenda for Medicine and Nursing," *New England Journal of Medicine* 307 (16 September 1982): 747–50.

31. Administrator's report, in the minutes of the Board of Trustees, CHH, 30 December 1952.

32. Idem, 23 February 1954.

33. Minutes of the Medical Staff Committee, Board of Trustees, CHH, 14 February 1949.

34. For a short overview of internships and residencies filled by foreign graduates, see Rashi Fein, *The Doctor Shortage: An Economic Diagnosis* (Washington, D.C.: Brookings Institution, 1967), 86–87.

35. Minutes of the Medical Staff Committee, Board of Trustees, CHH, 25 September 1951 and 28 December 1951. The officer of the day served as the house physician during the day and at night.

36. William B. Kouwenhoven, James R. Jude, and Guy G. Knickerbocker, "Closed Chest Cardiac Massage," *Journal of the American Medical Association* 173 (9 July 1960): 1064–67.

37. For descriptions of medical practice, see Temple Burling, Edith Lentz, and Robert N. Wilson, *The Give and Take in Hospitals* (New York: G. P. Putnam, 1956), 244–59; also Duff and Hollingshead, *Sickness and Society*, 133–36.

38. Rose Pinneo, telephone interview with Julie Fairman, 20 November 1991.

39. Strauss et al., *Social Organization*, 272, describe symbolic work as that which is accomplished when the power of actually doing the task takes precedence over skill, when the basis for allocation of a task is not related to the competence of the worker.

40. Joan Scott speaks to the importance of choices and the danger in minimizing choices constrained by gender and power issues in "History and Difference," in *Learning about Women: Gender, Politics, and Power*, ed. Jill Conway, Susan Bourque, and Joan Scott (Ann Arbor: University of Michigan Press, 1987), 93–118.

41. American Nurses Association Committee on Nursing Practice, "Closed Chest Cardiac Resuscitation . . . Professional and Legal Implications for Nurses," *American Journal of Nursing* 62 (May 1962): 94–95.

42. American Heart Association, "Closed-Chest Method of Cardiopulmonary Resuscitation," *Circulation* 31 (May 1965), reprinted in *American Journal of Nursing* 65 (May 1965): 105.

43. Minutes of the Subcommittee on Nursing, Medical Board, HUP, 8 May 1962, 19 December 1965.

44. Loretta C. Ford, "Nurse Practitioners: History of a New Idea and Predictions for the Future," in *Nursing in the 1980s: Crises, Opportunities, Challenges*, ed. Linda Aiken and Susan Gortner (Philadelphia: J. B. Lippincott, 1982), 231–47.

45. Aiken and Mechanic, "A Cooperative Agenda," 747–50.

46. Stein, Watts, and Howell, "Revisited," 546–49.

47. Patricia D'Antonio, "Tension at the Bedside," paper presented at the American Association of the History of Medicine, sixth annual meeting, Baltimore, Md., 1987.

48. Katherine H. Chavigny, "Medicine vs. Nursing, the RCT Proposal," *Nursing Management* 20 (August 1989): 38–40.

49. For an overview of commission findings, see National Joint Practice Commission, *Guidelines for Establishing Joint or Collaborative Practice in Hospitals: A Demonstration Project Directed by the National Joint Practice Commission, 1974* (Chicago: Nealy Printing, 1974). See also Fagin, "Collaboration," 295–303.

50. Fagin enumerates and describes the tensions in "Collaboration," 295–303.

51. Larson, interview, 7 September 1989.

52. Regina Bradley, interview with Julie Fairman, 31 January 1991, Chestnut Hill, Pa.

53. Donna Lee Bartram, interview with Joan Lynaugh at the American Association of Critical-Care Nurses Teaching Institute, May 1989, Atlanta, Ga.

54. Kinney, interview, May 1989.

55. Coser, *Life on the Ward*, 29–32; Fairman, "Watchful Vigilance," 56–60.

56. Kinney, interview, May 1989.

57. Kundrat and Bridal, interviews, 26 May 1989, and Kinney, interview, May 1989.

58. Kundrat, interview, 26 May 1989; Kinney, interview, May 1989. Kinney also adds that "maybe we were a lot to blame for the hierarchy that developed."

59. For examples, see Hughes, *Twenty Thousand Nurses*, 172–77; Duff and Hollingshead, *Sickness and Society*, 217–47.

60. The change in status is further supported by nurses' accounts of their estrangement from the hospital's nursing department, which thought they were practicing medicine (Kinney, interview, May 1989) and of requests from other nurses for instruction (Bridal, interview, 26 May 1989).

61. Fairman, "Watchful Vigilance," 56–60.

62. Ruth Jarousse, telephone interview with Julie Fairman, 1 February 1992.

63. Ibid.

64. Rose Pinneo, telephone interview with Julie Fairman, 17 November 1991.

65. Meltzer, Pinneo, and Kitchell, *Intensive Coronary Care*, i.

66. Strauss et al., *Social Organization,* 262–65. Robert Zussman ("Life in the Hospital: A Review," *Milbank Quarterly* 71 [1] [January 1993]: 167–85), on the other hand, believes the collective experience of patients is lost when they are conceptualized as part of the labor force, as Strauss et al. suggest.

67. Several studies examine the contribution of nurse-physician collaboration to patient outcome. One of the difficulties in assessing the studies is the numerous ways in which collaboration is defined and outcomes are measured. For examples, see M. Williams et al., "How Does the Team Approach to Outpatient Geriatric Evaluation Compare with Traditional Care: A Report of a Randomized Controlled Trial," *Journal of the American Geriatric Society* 35 (1987): 1071–79; B. Georgopoulos, "Organizational Structure and the Performance of Hospital Emergency Services," *Annals of Emergency Medicine* 14 (1985): 677–84; D. Kiz et al. "Examining Nursing Personnel Costs: Controlled Versus Non-Controlled Oral Analgesic Agents," *Journal of Nursing Administration* 19 (1) (1989):10–14; J. De-Fede, B. Dhanens, and N. Kelner, "Cost Benefits of Patient-Controlled Analgesia," *Nursing Management* 20 (5) (1989): 34–35. For an excellent overview, see also Fagin's analysis in "Collaboration," 295–303.

68. See William Knaus et al. "An Evaluation of Outcome from Intensive Care in Major Medical Centers," *Annals of Internal Medicine* 104 (March 1986): 410–18; Pam Mitchell et al. "American Association of Critical-Care Nurses Demonstration Project: Profile of Excellence in Critical Care Nursing," *Heart and Lung* 18 (1989): 219–37; Judith Baggs et al., "The Association between Interdisciplinary Collaboration and Patient Outcomes in a Medical Intensive Care Unit," *Heart and Lung* 21 (January 1992): 18–24.

Chapter 5: From General Duty Nurse to Specialist

1. Sydney Halpern, *American Pediatrics — The Social Dynamics of Professionalism, 1880–1980* (Berkeley: University of California Press, 1988), 159.

2. Shephard and Vaughan, interview, 15 August 1989. These founding members reported how difficult it was to train successfully in coronary care skills nurses who had been recruited involuntarily by their administrators to work in the units.

3. George Rosen, *The Specialization of Medicine* (New York: Froben Press, 1944; Chicago: Arno Press, 1972), 14.

4. For a more detailed history of the general expansion of nursing after World War II, see Joan Lynaugh and Barbara Brush, *American Nursing: From Hospitals to Health Systems* (Cambridge, Mass., and Oxford: Blackwell Publishing, 1996).

5. Shirley A. Smoyak, "Specialization in Nursing: From Then to Now," *Nursing Outlook* 24 (November 1976): 676–81.

6. In 1963, a study called *Toward Quality in Nursing* was commissioned and published by the U.S. Public Health Service. It called for federal dollars to underwrite the training of clinical specialists in nursing. This was

the blueprint for subsequent federal initiatives supporting higher education in nursing, i.e., the nurse training acts of 1964 and subsequent years.

7. Denise Geolot, "NP Education: Observations from a National Perspective," *Nursing Outlook* 35 (May/June 1987): 132–35.

8. National League for Nursing, *Nursing Data Review, 1989* (New York: National League for Nursing, 1990), 83.

9. Eugene Levine and Evelyn B. Moses, "Registered Nurses Today: A Statistical Profile," in *Nursing in the 1980s: Crises, Opportunities, Challenges,* ed. Linda Aiken and Susan Gortner (Philadelphia: J. B. Lippincott, 1982), 486. This number comes from the federal government and may be accurate, but there are wide variations in the counts of these specialty groups.

10. Data on master's and doctoral nurses are from U.S. Public Health Service, *Health, United States* (Washington, D.C.: GPO, 1988), and "RN Population Grows to a Million: Nurses Age But Work a Bit More," *American Journal of Nursing* (October 1994): 68.

11. Historian and physician Joel Howell's analysis of the medical story uses cardiology as an example ("The Changing Face of Twentieth-Century American Cardiology," *Annals of Internal Medicine* 105 [1986]: 772–82).

12. Claire Fagin, "Nursing's Pivotal Role in American Health Care," in Aiken and Gortner, *Nursing in the 1980s,* 459–502. This is one of several essays by this author linking the productivity of nurses and their safe-care results with the problems of financing U.S. health care. For a good discussion of "substitutive" nurse specialties, see Donna Diers, "Nurse Midwives and Nurse Anesthetists: The Cutting Edge of Specialist Practice," in *Charting Nursing's Future: Agenda for the Nineties,* ed. Linda Aiken and Claire Fagin (Philadelphia: J. B. Lippincott, 1991), 159–80.

13. Elting Morrison describes this as the preferred twentieth-century approach to change, i.e., the tendency to substitute testing of ideas and responsiveness for implementation of a grand design (*Man, Machines and Modern Times* [Cambridge: MIT Press, 1966], 212).

14. Mathy Mezey, "The Future of Primary Care and Nurse Practitioners," in *Nurses, Nurse Practitioners: The Evolution of Primary Care,* ed. Mathy D. Mezey and Diane O. McGivern (Boston and Toronto: Little, Brown and Co., 1986), 37–51.

15. Penny Vaughan, interview with Joan Lynaugh, 16 May 1989, Atlanta, Ga.

16. Donna Zschoche and Lillian E. Brown, "Intensive Care Nursing: Specialism, Junior Doctoring, or Just Nursing?" *American Journal of Nursing* 69 (November 1969): 2370–74.

17. "News of Note from Your A.A.C.N.," nos. 3, 5, and 9, archives, American Association of Critical-Care Nurses, Aliso Viejo, Calif.

18. In July of 1992, the AACN took over publishing responsibility for its journals, severing its twenty-year relationship with the C. V. Mosby Company of St. Louis. The new journal is called the *American Journal of Critical Care.* The original journal name may well have been a compromise selection of the nurses and physicians who originated it.

19. Public Relations Committee of the National Federation for Spe-

cialty Nursing Organizations, "NFSNO—The First Ten Years" (National Federation for Specialty Nursing Organizations, 1984), 2. Representatives of seventeen nursing organizations were invited; thirteen attended the meeting. The result was the NFSNO, a loosely organized group enabling continuing communication among the specialty organizations.

20. National Teaching Institutes Proceedings, 1974–1994, AACN Archives, Aliso Viejo, Calif.

21. AACN position statement, "Entry into Professional Nursing Practice, 1980," AACN Archives, Aliso Viejo, Calif.

22. AACN position statement, "Process for Addressing Practice, Political, and Professional Issues," approved by the board of directors in February 1983.

23. AACN position statement, "Resolution in Response to Action by the American Medical Association House of Delegates," October 1981. The AMA House of Delegates, fearing competition from nurses, decided to object to federal funding for nurse practitioner training and to allowing nurses to perform physical examinations and take patient histories in hospitals. Relationships between the specialty groups in medicine and nursing most concerned with critical care were always more amicable than relationships between the AACN and the AMA.

24. Pamela Mitchell, Sarah Armstrong, and Teri Forshee, "Excellence in Critical Care Nursing: It Can Be Done in the Cost-Containment Environment," (American Association of Critical-Care Nurses, Newport Beach, Calif., undated), AACN Archives, Aliso Viejo, Calif.; Sarah Armstrong, "The Cost of Nursing Excellence in Critical Care," *Journal of Nursing Administration* 21 (2) (February 1991): 27–33.

25. Patricia Benner, *From Novice to Expert—Excellence and Power in Clinical Nursing Practice* (Menlo Park, Calif.: Addison-Wesley, 1984). For this particular point, see Patricia Benner, Christine Tanner, and Carole Chesla, "From Beginner to Expert: Gaining a Differentiated Clinical World in Critical Care Nursing," *Advances in Nursing Science* 14 (1992): 13–28.

Chapter 6: At Century's End

1. Many people learn of cardiopulmonary resuscitation from television and have unrealistic expectations of its effectiveness. For a discussion of this issue, see S. J. Diem et al., "Cardiopulmonary Resuscitation on Television—Miracles and Misinformation," *New England Journal of Medicine* 334 (13 June 1996): 1578–82, and, in the same issue, Neal Baer, "Cardiopulmonary Resuscitation on Television," 1604–5.

2. An exceptional account of the need for making standard treatments widely available is Malcolm Gladwell's "Conquering the Coma," *New Yorker* (8 July 1996), which juxtaposes the family and personal stories of an assaulted, gravely injured Central Park jogger with the details on her treatment and the larger context in which her care was selected and given.

3. See SUPPORT Principle Investigators, "A Controlled Trial to Improve Care for Seriously Ill Hospitalized Patients," *Journal of the American*

Medical Association 274 (22–29 November 1995): 1591–98, for a discussion of the depth and seriousness of this reluctance to "enable" death. See also the annual report for 1995, "On Dying in America," of the Robert Wood Johnson Foundation, Princeton, N.J.

4. R. D. Berenson, *Intensive Care Units: Clinical Outcomes, Costs, and Decision Making*, Office of Technology Assessment, Health Technology Case Study no. 28 (Washington, D.C.: GPO, November 1984), 3.

5. For a thoughtful, early review, see William Knaus, Elizabeth Draper, and Douglas Wagner, "The Use of Intensive Care: New Research Initiatives and Their Implications for National Health Policy," *Milbank Memorial Fund Quarterly* 61 (Fall 1983): 561–82.

6. At the 1992 National Teaching Institute AACN president Wanda Roberts Johanson declared that "competence is fundamentally related to nurses' optimal contribution to mutually desired outcomes for patients and families." Wanda Roberts Johanson, presidential address, National Teaching Institute, 1992.

7. Grif Alspach, "Giving Voice to the Vision—Achieving the Patient-Driven System," *Critical Care Nurses*, supplement (June 1994): 2.

8. James R. Knickman, Mack Lipkin, Steven Finkler, Warren Thompson, and Joan Kiel, "The Potential for Using Non-Physicians to Compensate for the Reduced Availability of Residents," *Academic Medicine* 67 (July 1992): 429–37; Rosalyn J. Watts, Mary Jane Hanson, Kathleen Burke, Susan Gallagher, and Deborah Foster, "The Critical Care Nurse Practitioner: An Advanced Practice Role for the Critical Care Nurse," *Dimensions of Critical Care Nursing* 15 (January–February 1996): 48–56.

9. Linda Aiken, "Charting the Future of Hospital Nursing," *Image: Journal of Nursing Scholarship* 22 (Spring 1990): 72–78.

10. Wanda Roberts Johanson, presidential address, National Teaching Institute, 1992.

References

Piecing together the history of recent events from the documents and recollections of the participants in those events is fraught with difficulty and risk of error. The historical material to support this study was sequestered in hospital records, organization files, and the personal papers and memories of individuals. We list here the main collections from which we drew information and the names of those who shared their recollections with us. To assist others who will pursue this area of study we also list the professional and historical literature we found helpful. No such list of sources can be exhaustive as the subject of care of the critically ill attracts constant interest and investigation. The material we collected during this study will be available to scholars in the Center for the Study of the History of Nursing at the University of Pennsylvania.

Manuscript Collections

Archives, American Association of Critical-Care Nurses, Aliso Viejo, California

Annual reports, Board of Directors, 1970–1985.
Reports of subcommittees, 1970–1985.
Unpublished organizational histories.
Report of the Committee of the National Federation of Specialty Nursing, 1984.
Membership tabulations, 1970–1985.
AACN budgets, 1970–1985.
Membership publications and brochures.
Position statements, 1970–1985.
National Teaching Institute programs and planning papers.

Presidential addresses, 1970–1997.
Postcard collection, 1968.

Archives, Chestnut Hill Hospital, Hospital Library, Chestnut Hill

Annual reports, Board of Trustees, 1962–1967.
Bulletin, 1952–1965.
Medical Staff minutes, vol. 2, 1962–1967.
Minute books, Board of Trustees, 1945–1967.
Papers of Joseph C. Doane, "The Doane Report," 1948.
Papers of J. Don Miller, administrator.
Photograph file.
Records of CHH, minutes of various hospital committees and memoranda.
Telephone directories, various years.

Center for the Study of the History of Nursing, School of Nursing,
University of Pennsylvania, Philadelphia

HUP School of Nursing Collection

   Annual reports, Department of Nursing, 1964–1967.
   Reports, State Board of Nurse Examiners, 1950–1957.

Nadine Landis Collection, HUP

   Annual reports, Board of Managers, 1945–1967
   Logbook, Office of the Private-Duty Nurse Registrar.
   Photograph file.
   Annual reports, policy and procedure manuals, charts and graphs, Department of Nursing Service.
   HUP Memoranda books, minutes of standing and ad hoc committees.
   Records of the School of Nursing.
   National League for Nursing Accreditation survey and resurvey reports.

Mary Clymer Collection

   Student log, handwritten, 1887.

Historical Collection, College of Physicians of Philadelphia

Francis C. Wood Collection, 1950–1960 (uncataloged).

   Handwritten annual reports, Medical Department, HUP, 1950–1960.

Office of Post Graduate Education, Hospital of the
University of Pennsylvania, Philadelphia

Minutes, Department of Surgery, 1945–1970.
Morbidity and mortality reports, 1945–1965.

Office of Medical Affairs, Hospital of the
University of Pennsylvania, Philadelphia

Minutes, Medical Board, 1946–1970.
Reports, Delaware Valley Hospital Council, 1964–1967.

Temple University, Urban Archives Collection, Philadelphia

Evening Bulletin Collection, 1957.

Interviews

Hospital of the University of Pennsylvania

Nurses: Betty Lou Bridal, Linda Capone, Patricia Davies, Peggy Fuhs, Mary Conneely Gorka, Beth Helwig, Mary Holbey, Karen Krietz Johnson, Nadine Landis, Mary Alice Musser, Patricia Mynaugh, Edna Reilly, Mary Rieser, Maureen O'Hern, Karen Moore Schaeffer, and Gloria Woolever Kundrat.
Physicians: Clyde Barker, John Helwig Jr., Jonathan Rhoads, Brooke Roberts, John Sayen, Truman Schnable, Cletus Schwegman, and Francis C. Wood.
Administrators: Ralph Perkins and Kenneth Wenrich.

Chestnut Hill Hospital

Nurses: Laura Mae Beery, Regina Bradley, Jane Danihel, Maureen Hamilton, Ruth Jarousse, Julie McGann, and Helen Richards.
Physicians: Thomas Clark, Clifford Loew, Charles T. Lee, and Henry Lee.
Administrator: J. Don Miller.

Intensive and Coronary Care Nursing and the American
Association of Critical-Care Nurses

Diane Adler, Donna Lee Bartram, Joanne Disch, Kathleen Dracup, Jeannette Hartshorn, Mairead Hickey, Marguerite Kinney, Rebecca Kuhn,

Eleanor Lambertsen, Rosalie Hammerschmidt Lanius, Cheryl Larson, Sally Millar, Pamela Mitchell, Rose Pinneo, Wanda Salas, Linda Samson, Linda Searles, Barbara Siebelt, Norma Shephard, Penny Vaughn, and Patricia Yates.

Books and Journals

General Nursing and Hospitals

Abdellah, Faye, Irene L. Beland, Almeda Martin, and Ruth V. Matheney, eds. *Patient-Centered Approaches to Nursing.* New York: Macmillan Co., 1960.

Aiken, Linda. "Charting the Future of Hospital Nursing." *Image: Journal of Nursing Scholarship* 22 (Spring 1990): 72–78.

Aiken, Linda, and Claire Fagin, eds. *Charting Nursing's Future: Agenda for the Nineties.* Philadelphia: J. B. Lippincott, 1991.

Aiken, Linda, and Susan Gortner, eds. *Nursing in the 1980s: Crises, Opportunities, Challenges.* Philadelphia: J. B. Lippincott, 1982.

Aiken, Linda, and David Mechanic. "A Cooperative Agenda for Medicine and Nursing." *New England Journal of Medicine* 307 (16 September 1982): 747–50.

Alcott, Louisa May. *Hospital Sketches.* Boston: James Redpath, 1863.

Allen, Rex W. "Designed for Nursing." *American Journal of Nursing* 64 (February 1964): 91.

American Association of Critical-Care Nurses, Kansas City chapter. *Kansas City Media Award Interviews.* Videotape, 1987.

American Hospital Association. "Annual Guide Issue." *Hospitals.* 1948–1970.

American Nurses' Association. *Facts About Nursing: A Statistical Summary.* New York: American Nurses' Association, 1950–1970.

American Nurses' Association Committee on Nursing Practice. "Closed Chest Cardiac Resuscitation . . . Professional and Legal Implications for Nurses." *American Journal of Nursing* 62 (May 1962): 94–95.

Aydelotte, Myrtle K. *Survey of Hospital Nursing Services.* New York: National League for Nursing, 1968.

Bankert, Marian. *Watchful Care: A History of America's Nurse Anesthetists.* New York: Continuum, 1989.

Barrett, Jean. *Ward Management and Teaching.* New York: Appleton-Century-Crofts, 1954.

Bates, Barbara. *Bargaining for Life: A Social History of Tuberculosis, 1876–1938.* Philadelphia: University of Pennsylvania Press, 1992.

Beck, Claude, and David S. Leighninger. "Death After a Clean Bill of Health." *Journal of the American Medical Association* 174 (10 September 1960): 117–35.

Belknap, Ivan, and John G. Steinle. *The Community and Its Hospitals: A Comparative Analysis.* Syracuse, N.Y.: Syracuse University Press, 1963.

Benner, Patricia. *From Novice to Expert: Excellence and Power in Clinical Nursing Practice*. Menlo Park, Calif.: Addison-Wesley, 1984.

Benner, Patricia, Christine Tanner, and Carole Chesla. "From Beginner to Expert: Gaining a Differentiated Clinical World in Critical Care Nursing." *Advances in Nursing Science* 14 (1992): 13–28.

Bosk, Charles. *Forgive and Remember: Managing Medical Failure*. Chicago: University of Chicago Press, 1979.

Brannon, Robert. *Intensifying Care: The Hospital Industry, Professionalization, and the Reorganization of the Nursing Labor Process*. Amityville, N.Y.: Baywood Publishing Co., 1944.

Bressler, Marvin, and William Kephart. *Career Dynamics: A Survey of Selected Aspects of the Nursing Profession*. Harrisburg: Pennsylvania Nurses' Association, 1955.

——. *Career Dynamics, Philadelphia PA, University of Pennsylvania*. Philadelphia: Pennsylvania Nurses' Association, 1955.

Bridgman, Margaret. *Collegiate Education for Nursing*. New York: Russell Sage Foundation, 1953.

Brown, Esther Lucile. *Nursing for the Future: A Report for the National Nursing Council*. New York: Russell Sage Foundation, 1948.

Brush, Barbara. "A Marriage of Convenience: Group Nursing in United States Hospitals, 1918–1930." Unpublished manuscript, 16 April 1991.

Bullock, Robert P. *What Do Nurses Think of Their Profession?* Columbus: Ohio State University Research Foundation, 1954.

Burling, Temple, Edith Lentz, and Robert N. Wilson. *The Give and Take in Hospitals*. New York: G. P. Putnam, 1956.

Butter, Irene. "The Supply of Nurses—Its Responsiveness to Economic Incentives." In *Hospital Nursing Shortage: Crisis or Illusion*, 19–48. Ann Arbor: University of Michigan Press, 1967.

"Care of Hypodermic Needles and Syringes." *American Journal of Nursing* 52 (March 1952): 297.

Carnevali, Doris, and Nola Smith Sheldon. "How Early Ambulation Affects Nursing Service." *American Journal of Nursing* 52 (August 1952): 954–56.

Chafe, William H. *The American Woman: Her Changing Social, Economic and Political Roles, 1920–1970*. London and Oxford: Oxford University Press, 1972.

"Changes in Nursing from 1938 to 1953." *Nursing Research* 5 (October 1956): 85–86.

Chavigny, Katherine H. "Medicine vs. Nursing, the RCT Proposal." *Nursing Management* 20 (August 1989): 38–40.

Clark, Clifford E. "Ranch-House Suburbia: Ideals and Realities." In *Recasting America: Culture and Politics in the Age of Cold War*, edited by Larry May, 179–90. Chicago: University of Chicago Press, 1989.

Corner, George W. *Two Centuries of Medicine: A History of the School of Medicine, University of Pennsylvania*. Philadelphia: J. B. Lippincott Co., 1965.

Coser, Rose Laub. *Life on the Ward*. East Lansing: Michigan State University Press, 1962.

Coser, Rose L., H. Becker, B. Greer, E. Hughes, and A. Strauss. *Boys in*

White: Student Cultures in Medical Schools. Chicago: University of Chicago Press, 1961.

Coughlin, Robert E. "Hospital Complex Analysis: An Approach to Analysis for Planning a Metropolitan System of Service Facilities." Ph.D. diss., University of Pennsylvania, 1964.

Curran, Jean A., and Helen L. Bunge. *Better Nursing: A Study of Nursing Care and Education in Washington.* Seattle: University of Washington Press, 1951.

Davies, Celia. "Introduction: The Contemporary Challenge in Nursing History." In *Rewriting Nursing History,* edited by Celia Davies, 10–11. London: Croom Helm, 1980.

D'Antonio, Patricia. "Tension at the Bedside." Paper presented at the American Association of the History of Medicine, Sixth Annual Meeting, Baltimore, Md., 1987.

DeFede, J., B. Dhanens, and N. Kelner. "Cost Benefits of Patient-Controlled Analgesia." *Nursing Management* 20 (5) (1989): 34–35.

Dennison, Claire. "Maintaining the Quality of Nursing Service in the Emergency Room." *American Journal of Nursing* 42 (July 1942): 774.

Diers, Donna. "Nurse Midwives and Nurse Anesthetists: The Cutting Edge of Specialist Practice." In *Charting Nursing's Future: Agenda for the Nineties,* edited by Linda Aiken and Claire Fagin, 159–80. Philadelphia: J. B. Lippincott, 1991.

Duff, Raymond S., and August B. Hollinghead. *Sickness and Society.* New York: Harper and Row, 1968.

Fagin, Claire M. "Collaboration Between Nurses and Physicians: No Longer a Choice." *Academic Medicine* 67 (May 1992): 295–303.

Fagin, Claire. "Nursing's Pivotal Role in American Health Care." In *Nursing in the 1980s: Crises, Opportunities, Challenges,* edited by Linda Aiken and Susan Gortner, 459–502. Philadelphia: Lippincott.

Fairman, Julie. "When the Emergency Was Routine." Presented at the annual conference of the American Association for the History of Nursing, Cincinnati, Ohio, 1988.

Fein, Rashi. *The Doctor Shortage: An Economic Diagnosis.* Washington, D.C.: Brookings Institution, 1967.

Field, Hermann H., John A. Hanson, Constantine J. Karalis, Donald A. Kennedy, Stanley Lippert, and Paul G. Ronco, eds. *Evaluation of Hospital Design: A Holistic Approach.* Boston: Tufts–New England Medical Center, 1971.

Flood, Marilyn. "Crossroads Revisited." *Nursing Research* 39 (November/December 1990): 380–81.

———. "The Troubling Expedient: General Staff Nursing in the United States Hospitals in the 1930s: A Means to Institutional, Educational and Personal Ends." Ph.D. diss., University of California, Berkeley, 1981.

Ford, Loretta C. "Nurse Practitioners: History of a New Idea and Predictions for the Future." In *Nursing in the 1980s: Crises, Opportunities, Challenges,* edited by Linda Aiken and Susan Gortner, 231–47. Philadelphia: J. B. Lippincott, 1982.

Ford, Thomas R., and Diane D. Stephenson. *Institutional Nurses: Roles, Re-*

lationships, and Attitudes in Three Alabama Hospitals. University: University of Alabama Press, 1954.

Fox, Renee. "Training for Uncertainty." In *The Student-Physician: Introductory Studies in the Sociology of Medical Education,* edited by Robert Merton, George Reader, and Patricia Kendall, 207–41. Cambridge, Mass.: Harvard University Press, 1957.

Fox, Renee, and Judith Swarez. *The Courage to Fail: A Social View of Organ Transplantation and Dialysis.* Chicago: University of Chicago Press, 1974.

Frieson, Gordon. "Integrated Communication Through Construction." *Hospital Progress* 7 (August 1960): 64–67.

Galambos, Louis G., and Joseph Pratt. *The Rise of the Corporate Commonwealth: United States Business and Public Policy in the Twentieth Century.* New York: Basic Books, 1988.

Geolot, Denise. "NP Education: Observations from a National Perspective." *Nursing Outlook* 35 (May/June 1987): 132–35.

George, F. L., and D. Popovitch. "What About a Voice Intercom System?" *Hospitals* 28 (February 1954): 80.

Georgopoulos, B. "Organizational Structure and the Performance of Hospital Emergency Services." *Annals of Emergency Medicine* 14 (1985): 677–84.

Ginzberg, Eli G. *A Program for the Nursing Profession.* New York: Macmillan Co., 1948.

Governmental Research Center, University of Kansas. *The Study of Activities of Registered Professional Nurses in Small Kansas Hospitals.* Lawrence: University of Kansas, 1953.

Halpern, Sydney. *American Pediatrics: The Social Dynamics of Professionalism, 1880–1980.* Berkeley: University of California Press, 1988.

Health Insurance Institute. *Source Book of Health Insurance Data, 1963.* New York: The Institute, 1963.

Hirst, J. Willis, and R. Bruce Logue, eds. *The Heart.* New York: McGraw-Hill, 1966.

Hughes, Everett C. *Men and Their Work.* London: Free Press of Glencoe, 1958.

Hughes, Everett C., Helen MacGill Hughes, and Irwin Deutscher. *Twenty Thousand Nurses Tell Their Story.* Philadelphia: J. B. Lippincott, 1958.

Kalisch, Phillip, and Beatrice Kalisch. *The Advance of American Nursing,* 2d ed. Boston and Toronto: Little, Brown and Co., 1986.

Kessler-Harris, Alice. *Out to Work: A History of Wage-Earning Women in the United States.* New York: Oxford University Press, 1982.

Kiz, D., M. McCartney, J. Kissick, and R. Townsend. "Examining Nursing Personnel Costs: Controlled Versus Non-Controlled Oral Analgesic Agents." *Journal of Nursing Administration* 19 (1) (1989): 10–14.

Klarman, Herbert E. *The Economics of Health.* New York: Columbia University Press, 1965.

Knickman, James R., Mack Lipkin, Steven Finkler, Warren Thompson, and Joan Kiel. "The Potential for Using Non-Physicians to Compensate for the Reduced Availability of Residents." *Academic Medicine* 67 (July 1992): 429–37.

Lambertsen, Eleanor C. *Nursing Team Organization and Function.* New York: Columbia University Teachers College, 1953.

Leone, Lucile Petry, and Louis Block. *Cost Analysis for Schools of Nursing.* Washington, D.C.: U.S. Public Health Service, 1947.

Levine, Eugene. "Turnover Among Nursing Personnel in General Hospitals." *Hospitals* 31 (1 September 1957): 50–53, 138–40.

Levine, Eugene, and Evelyn B. Moses. "Registered Nurses Today: A Statistical Profile." In *Nursing in the 1980s: Crises, Opportunities, Challenges,* edited by Linda Aiken and Susan Gortner. Philadelphia: J. B. Lippincott, 1982.

Lundberg, Ferdinand, and Marynia Farnham. *Modern Women: The Lost Sex.* New York: Harper and Brothers, 1947.

Lynaugh, Joan. "Narrow Passageways: Nurses and Physicians in Conflict and Concert Since 1875." In *The Physician as Captain of the Ship: A Critical Reappraisal,* edited by Nancy King, Larry Churchill, and Alan Cross. Boston: D. Reidel, 1988.

McBride, David. *Integrating the City of Medicine: Blacks in Philadelphia Health Care, 1910–1965.* Philadelphia: Temple University Press, 1989.

Mead, Margaret. *Male and Female.* New York: Morrow, 1947.

Melosh, Barbara. "More Than 'The Physician's Hand': Skill and Authority in Twentieth-Century Nursing." In *Women and Health in America,* edited by Judith Walzer Leavitt, 482–96. Madison: University of Wisconsin Press, 1984.

———. *The Physician's Hand: Work Culture and Conflict in American Nursing.* Philadelphia: Temple University Press, 1982.

Mezey, Mathy. "The Future of Primary Care and Nurse Practitioners." In *Nurses, Nurse Practitioners: The Evolution of Primary Care,* edited by Mathy D. Mezey and Diane O. McGivern, 37–51. Boston and Toronto: Little, Brown and Co., 1986.

National Academy of Engineering. *Costs of Health Care Facilities.* Washington, D.C.: National Academy of Science, 1968.

National Joint Practice Commission. *Guidelines for Establishing Joint or Collaborative Practice in Hospitals: A Demonstration Project Directed by the National Joint Practice Commission, 1974.* Chicago: Nealy Printing, 1974.

National League for Nursing. *Nursing Data Review, 1989.* New York: National League for Nursing, 1990.

———. *Report on Hospital Schools of Nursing, 1957.* New York: NLN, 1959.

Newcomb, Dorothy Perkins. *The Team Plan: A Manual for Nursing Service Administrators.* New York: G. P. Putnam, 1953.

New York University. *A Study of Nursing Functions in Twelve Hospitals in the State of New York.* New York: New York University, 1952.

Nightingale, Florence. *Notes on Hospitals.* 3d ed. New York: Longman, Green, Longman, Roberts, and Green, 1863.

Pennsylvania Nurses' Association. *Employment Standards for Pennsylvania Nurses.* Harrisburg: Pennsylvania Nurses Association, 1958 and 1962.

Perrow, Charles. "Goals and Power Structures: A Historical Case Study." In *The Hospital in Modern Society,* edited by Elliot Friedson, 143–44. London: Collier, 1963.

Pfefferkorn, Blanche, and Charles A. Rovetts. *Administrative Cost Analysis for Nursing Service and Nursing Education.* New York: American Hospital Association and the National League of Nursing Education, 1940.

Philadelphia General Hospital School of Nursing. *Nursing Procedures.* Philadelphia: Philadelphia General Hospital, 1954.

Pollak, Otto, Charles F. Westoff, and Marvin Bressler. *Pennsylvania Pilot Study of Nursing Functions.* Harrisburg: Pennsylvania Nurses' Association, 1953.

Prescott, Patricia, and Sally Bowen. "Physician-Nurse Relationships." *Annals of Internal Medicine* 103 (1) (July 1985): 127–33.

President's Commission on the Health Needs of the Nation. *Building America's Health.* Vol. 3. Washington, D.C.: GPO, 1953.

Price, Elmina Mary. *Learning Needs of Registered Nurses.* New York: Teachers College Press, 1967.

Reissman, Leonard, and John H. Rohrer, *Change and Dilemma in the Nursing Profession.* New York: G. P. Putnam, 1957.

Reverby, Susan. *Ordered to Care: The Dilemma of American Nursing, 1850–1945.* Cambridge: Cambridge University Press, 1987.

"RN Population Grows to a Million: Nurses Age but Work a Bit More." *American Journal of Nursing* (October 1994): 68.

Roberts, Mary M. *American Nursing: History and Interpretation.* New York: Macmillan Co., 1954.

Rosen, George. *The Specialization of Medicine.* New York: Froben Press, 1944; Chicago: Arno Press, 1972.

Rosenberg, Charles. *The Care of Strangers: The Rise of America's Hospital System.* New York: Basic Books, 1987.

Ross, Mary. "Private Life or Private Duty for the R.N." *Survey* 60 (February 1921): 549–52.

Scott, Joan. "History and Difference." In *Learning About Women: Gender, Politics, and Power,* edited by Jill Conway, Susan Bourque, and Joan Scott, 93–118. Ann Arbor: University of Michigan Press, 1987.

Scott, Joan Wallach. "The Problem of Invisibility." In *Retrieving Women's History: Changing Perceptions of the Role of Women in Politics and Society,* edited by S. J. Kleinberg, 5–29. New York: Berg Publishers, 1988.

Scottish Home and Health Department. *The Falkirk Ward.* Vol. 4. Edinburgh: Author, 1969.

Smoyak, Shirley A. "Specialization in Nursing: From Then to Now." *Nursing Outlook* 24 (November 1976): 676–81.

Sobol, Marion G. "Commitment to Work." In *The Employed Mother in America,* edited by Ivan F. Ny and Lois W. Hoffman, 40–63. Chicago: Rand McNally, 1963.

Somers, Herman M., and Anne R. Somers. *Doctors, Patients and Health Insurance.* Washington, D.C.: Brookings Institute, 1961.

Sommer, Robert. "Personal Space." *Canadian Architect* 5 (February 1960): 76–80.

Spohn, Roberta. "Some Facts About the Nursing 'Shortage.'" *American Journal of Nursing* 54 (July 1954): 865–66.

Starr, Paul. *The Social Transformation of American Medicine.* New York: Basic Books, 1982.

Stein, Leonard. "The Doctor-Nurse Game." *Archives of General Psychiatry* 16 (June 1967): 699–703.

Stein, Leonard, David Watts, and Timothy Howell. "The Doctor-Nurse Game Revisited" *New England Journal of Medicine* 322 (22 February 1990): 546–49.

Stevens, Rosemary. *In Sickness and in Wealth: American Hospitals in the Twentieth Century.* New York: Basic Books, 1989.

———. "A Poor Sort of Memory: Voluntary Hospital and Government Before the Depression." *Milbank Memorial Fund Quarterly* 60 (1982): 551–84.

Stewart, Donald, and Christine E. Needham. *The General Duty Nurse.* Fayetteville: University of Arkansas, 1955.

Stewart, Isabel Maitland. *The Education of Nurses: Historical Foundations and Modern Trends.* New York: Macmillan Co., 1945.

Stewart, William H. "The Surgeon General Looks at Nursing." *American Journal of Nursing* 67 (January 1967): 65.

Strauss, Anselm, Shizuko Fagerhaugh, Barbara Suczek, and Carolyn Wiener. *Social Organization of Medical Work.* Chicago: University of Chicago Press, 1985.

Strauss, Anselm, Leonard Schatzman, Danuta Ehrlich, Rue Bucher, and Melvin Sabshin. "The Hospital and Its Negotiated Order." In *Profession of Medicine: A Study of the Sociology of Applied Knowledge,* edited by Eliot Friedson, 147–69. New York: Atherton Press, 1970.

Teaford, Jon C. *The Twentieth-Century American City: Problem, Promise, and Reality,* Baltimore: Johns Hopkins University Press, 1986.

Testoff, Arthur, Eugene Levine, and Stanley E. Siegel. "The Part-Time Nurse." *American Journal of Nursing* (January 1964): 88–89.

Thompson, John D. "How Many Oxygen Outlets?" *Modern Hospital* 92 (January 1959): 116–22.

Thompson, John D., and Grace Goldin. *The Hospital: A Social and Architectural History.* New Haven, Conn.: Yale University Press, 1975.

"Three Meetings and Their Messages." *Charities* II (25) (week ending 19 December 1903): 580.

"Twenty Studies of Nursing Functions." *American Journal of Nursing* 54 (November 1954): 1378–82.

U.S. Congress. Senate Committee on Labor and Public Welfare. *Study of Health Facilities Construction Costs.* Washington, D.C.: GPO, 1972.

U.S. Department of Health, Education, and Welfare. *Health Manpower Source Book.* Section 2, revised. Washington, D.C.: GPO, 1965.

———. Division of Regional Medical Programs. *Guidelines—Regional Medical Programs.* Washington, D.C.: GPO, 1968 (revised).

———. Public Health Service. *Elements of Progressive Patient Care.* Washington, D.C.: Department of Health, Education, and Welfare, 1959, microfiche.

———. Public Health Service. *Medical Care Financing and Utilization: Source*

Book of Data Through 1961. Health Economics Series no. 1. Washington, D.C.: GPO, 1962.

————. Public Health Service. *Nursing Resources: A Progress Report of the Program of the Division of Nursing Resources.* Prepared under the direction of Apollonia O. Adams, PHS pub. no. 551. Washington, D.C.: GPO, 1958.

————. Public Health Service. *Towards Quality in Nursing—Needs and Goals.* Public Health Service Publication No. 992. Washington, D.C.: GPO, 1963.

————. Public Health Service. Division of Nursing Resources. *For Better Nursing in Michigan: A Survey of Needs and Resources.* Detroit, Mich.: Cunningham Drug Co. Foundation, 1954.

U.S. Department of Labor. Women's Bureau. "The Outlook for Women in Professional Nursing Occupations." *Bulletin of the Womens' Bureau.* 203–3 revised. Washington, D.C.: GPO, 1953.

U.S. Public Health Service. *Health, United States.* Washington, D.C.: GPO, 1988.

————. "Hospital Profiles: A Decade of Change, 1953–1962." *Modern Hospital* 102, 2 (February 1964): 92–101.

————. Division of Nursing Resources. *How to Study Nursing Activities in a Patient Unit.* Pub. no. 370. Washington, D.C.: GPO, 1954.

————. Federal Security Agency. *Blue Cross and Medical Service Plans.* By Louis S. Reed. Washington, D.C.: GPO, 1947.

————. Federal Security Agency. *The Cadet Nurse Corp, 1943–1948.* Pub. no. 38. Washington, D.C.: GPO, 1950.

————. Federal Security Agencies. Division of Nursing Resources. *The Washington Nursing Survey.* Washington, D.C.: GPO, 1950.

University of California School of Nursing. *A Functional Analysis of Nursing Service.* San Francisco: University of California, 1950.

Washington State Nurses' Association. *Nursing Functions Study: An Analysis of the Nursing Activities of a Medical Service.* Seattle: Washington State Nurses' Association, 1953.

Watts, Rosalyn J., Mary Jane Hanson, Kathleen Burke, Susan Gallagher, and Deborah Foster. "The Critical Care Nurse Practitioner: An Advanced Practice Role for the Critical Care Nurse." *Dimensions of Critical Care Nursing* 15 (January–February 1996): 48–56.

Weeks, Lewis, ed. *Faye Abdellah in First Person: An Oral History.* Chicago: American Hospital Association Research and Educational Trust, 1983.

Weiss, Robert, and Nancy Samuelson. "Social Roles of American Women: Their Contribution to a Sense of Usefulness and Importance." *Journal of Marriage and the Family* 20 (November 1958): 358–66.

West, Margaret, and Christy Hawkins. *Nursing Schools at the Mid-Century.* New York: National Committee for the Improvement of Nursing Services, 1950.

Williams, M., T. Williams, J. Zimmer, W. Hall, M. Podgorski. "How Does the Team Approach to Outpatient Geriatric Evaluation Compare with Traditional Care? A Report of a Randomized Controlled Trial." *Journal of the American Geriatric Society* 35 (1987).

Wolf, Morris. "Practical Nurses—Letters to the Editor." *American Journal of Nursing* 52 (March 1952): 26.

Wolf, Zane Robinson. *Nurses' Work, The Sacred and the Profane.* Philadelphia: University of Pennsylvania Press, 1988.

Zussman, Robert. "Life in the Hospital: A Review." *Milbank Quarterly* 71 (1) (January 1993): 167–85.

Intensive Care Units and Recovery Rooms

Abdellah, Faye G. "Progressive Patient Care." *American Journal of Nursing* 59 (May 1959): 649–55.

———. "Progressive Patient Care—A Challenge for Nursing." *Hospital Management* (June 1960): 102–6, 135.

Abdellah Faye G., and E. Josephine Strachan. "Progressive Patient Care." *American Journal of Nursing* 59 (May, 1959): 649–55.

Ad Hoc Committee of the Harvard Medical School to Examine the Definition of Brain Death. "A Definition of Irreversible Coma." *Journal of the American Medical Association* 205 (5 August 1968): 85–88.

Alspach, Grif. "Giving Voice to the Vision—Achieving the Patient-Driven System." *Critical Care Nurses,* supplement (June 1994): 2.

Aydelotte, Myrtle Kitchell, and Marie E. Tener. *An Investigation of the Relation Between Nursing Activity and Patient Welfare.* Iowa City: State University of Iowa, 1960.

Ayers, Steven M. "Introduction: Critical-Care Medicine." In *Major Issues in Critical-Care Medicine,* edited by J. E. Parillo and Steven Ayers, xvii–xx. Baltimore: Wilkins and Wilkins, 1984.

Baggs, Judith, Sheila Ryan, Charles Phelps, Franklin Richeson, and Jean Johnson. "The Association Between Interdisciplinary Collaboration and Patient Outcomes in a Medical Intensive Care Unit." *Heart and Lung* 21 (January 1992): 18–24.

Barton, Jane. "Round the Clock Nursing or Self-Service: Patient Care Is Based on the Medical Need." *Modern Hospital* 88 (June 1957): 51–56.

Beardsley, J. Murray, J. Robert Brown, and Carmine J. Capalbo. "Centralized Treatment for Seriously Ill Surgical Patients." *Journal of the American Medical Association* 162 (6 October 1958): 544–47.

Beardsley J. Murray, and Florence Carvisiglia. "A Special Care Ward for Surgical Patients." *Nursing World* 131 (March 1957): 11.

Bell, Elizabeth A. "Special Nursing Unit Relieves the Strain." *Modern Hospital* 83 (November 1954): 74–75.

Bryan-Brown, Christopher W., and Kathleen Dracup. "1993: A Precarious Year for Critical Care." *American Journal of Critical Care* 2 (November 1993): 434–35.

Cadmus, Robert R. "Intensive Care Reaches Silver Anniversary." *Hospitals* 54 (16 January 1980): 98–102.

———. "Special Care for the Critical Case." *Hospitals* 28 (September 1954): 65.

Charbon, H., and H. M. Livingstone. "Planning a Recovery Room for Adequate Postoperative Care." *Hospitals* 23 (August 1949): 35–38.

Claussen, Esther. "Categorization of Patients According to Nursing Care Needs." *Military Medicine* 116 (March 1955): 214.

Clipson, Colin W., and Joseph J. Wehrer. *Planning for Cardiac Care: A Guide to the Planning and Design of Cardiac Care Facilities.* Ann Arbor, Mich.: Health Administration Press, 1973.

Conboy, Catherine F. "A Recovery Room." *American Journal of Nursing* 47 (October 1947): 686–87.

Day, Hughes W. "History of Coronary Units." *American Journal of Cardiology* 30 (September 1972): 405–6.

Dunn, Florence, and Miriam G. Shupp. "The Recovery Room: A Wartime Economy." *American Journal of Nursing* 49 (March 1943): 136–37.

Fairman, Julie. "Watchful Vigilance: Nursing Care, Technology, and the Development of Intensive Care Units." *Nursing Research* 41 (January/February 1992): 56–60.

Fuhs, Margaret, Mary Rieser, and Delores Brisbon. "Nursing in a Respiratory Intensive Care Unit." *Chest* 62 (August 1972, supplement): 14s–18s.

Harvey, A. McGehee. "Neurosurgical Genius: Walter Edward Dandy." *Hopkins Medicine* 135 (November 1974): 364–65.

Haver, Harry T., and Harry T. Haver Jr. "Subrecovery Unit Solved a Familiar Problem for This Hospital." *Hospitals* 31 (October 1957): 47–48.

Hilberman, Mark. "The Evolution of Intensive Care Units." *Critical Care Medicine* 3 (1975): 159–65.

Hook, Edward W., Christy A. Horton, and Dennis R. Schaberg. "Failure of Intensive Care Unit Support to Influence Mortality from Pneumococcal Bacteremia." *Journal of the American Medical Association* 249 (25 February 1983): 1055–57.

Ibsen, Bjorn. "The Anesthetists' Viewpoint on Treatment of Respiratory Complications in Poliomyelitis During the Epidemic in Copenhagen." *Proceedings of the Royal Society of Medicine* 47 (1954): 72–80.

"Intensive Care Unit." *Lankenau Magazine* (1961): 12.

Knaus, William, Elizabeth Draper, and Douglas Wagner. "The Use of Intensive Care: New Research Initiatives and Their Implications for National Health Policy." *Milbank Memorial Fund Quarterly* 61 (Fall 1983): 561–82.

Knaus, William A., Elizabeth A. Draper, Douglas P. Wagner, and Jack E. Zimmerman. "An Evaluation of Outcome from Intensive Care in Major Medical Centers." *Annals of Internal Medicine* 104 (March 1986): 410–18.

Knaus, William A., and George E. Thibault. "Intensive Care Units Today." In *Critical Issues in Medical Technology,* edited by Barbara J. McNeil and Ernest G. Cravalho, 195–98. Boston: Auburn House, 1982.

Krohn, Eleanor Dorothy. "Study to Determine the Knowledge, Understanding, and Skills Needed by the Professional Nurse in the Intensive Care Unit." Master's thesis, University of Colorado, 1960.

Lassen, H. C. "Preliminary Report on the 1952 Epidemic of Poliomyelitis in Copenhagen." *Lancet* 1 (1960): 37–40.

Last, Theodore. "Concentrating on the Critically Ill." *Hospitals* 86 (June 1956): 69–71.

Leon, Sr. Agnes. "Postanesthetic and Postoperative Recovery Units." *American Journal of Nursing* 52 (April 1952): 430–32.

Lockward, Howard J., Lane Giddings, and Edward J. Thoms. "Progressive Patient Care: A Preliminary Report." *Journal of the American Medical Association* 172 (9 January 1960): 132–37.

Lynaugh, Joan. "Critical Care Nursing: Past, Present, and Future." Speech to the Pennsylvania Chapter of the American Association of Critical Care Nurses, May 1991, Lankenau Hospital, Philadelphia.

———. "Four Hundred Postcards." *Nursing Research* 39 (July/August 1990): 252–53.

Lynaugh, Joan, and Barbara Brush. *American Nursing: From Hospitals to Health Systems.* Cambridge, Mass., and Oxford: Blackwell Publishing, 1996.

Manfreda, Emma P. "Polio Nursing, 1952." *Newsletter of the American Association for the History of Nursing* 30 (Spring 1991): 6–7.

Matkowski, Annette. "James William White, M.D., Ph.D., LL.D." In *Annual Report of the Harrison Department of Surgical Research and the Department of Surgery*, 5. Philadelphia, Pa., June 1971.

McClenahan, William U. *G.P.* Philadelphia: Dorrance and Co., 1974.

Meltzer, Lawrence E., Rose Pinneo, and J. Roderick Kitchell. *Intensive Coronary Care—A Manual for Nurses.* Philadelphia: CCU Fund, 1965.

Miller, J. Don. "The Critical Care Unit in a 134-Bed Hospital." *Hospitals* 30 (16 October 1956): 46–47, 96.

———. "Report on New Nursing Service." *Philadelphia Medicine* (18 March 1955): 935.

Mitchell, Pam, Sarah Armstrong, Teri Forshee Simpson, Margaret Nield, and Martha Lentz. "American Association of Critical-Care Nurses Demonstration Project: Profile of Excellence in Critical Care Nursing." *Heart and Lung* 18 (1989): 219–37.

Mosenthal, William, and David D. Boyd. "Special Unit Saves Lives, Nurses, Money." *Modern Hospital* 89 (December 1957): 83–86.

Nocella, Rosemary, Polly Barrick, and Lucy Fort. "The Evolution of Critical Care Nursing." Photocopy. North Carolina Memorial Hospital, Chapel Hill.

Parillo, Joseph E., and Stephen M. Ayers, eds. *Major Issues in Critical Care Medicine.* Baltimore: Williams and Wilkins, 1986.

Office of Technology Assessment. *Intensive Care Units: Clinical Outcomes, Costs, and Decision Making.* By R. D. Berenson. Health Technology Case Study no. 28. Washington, D.C.: GPO, November 1984.

Rieser, Mary, E. Carmelite, and Martha Taylor. "Intensive Care Nursing." In *Advanced Concepts in Clinical Nursing*, edited by Kay Kintzel, 68–80. Philadelphia: J. B. Lippincott, 1971.

Robinson, Edward. "Determining Nursing Staffing Patterns for an Intensive Care Unit, Part III: Conclusions and Recommendations." *Hospital Topics* (December 1960): 47–56, 64.

Russell, Louise B. *Technology in Hospitals: Medical Advances and Their Diffu-sion.* Washington, D.C.: Brookings Institution, 1979.

Ruth, Henry R., Frederick Haugen, and Dwight Grove. "Anesthesia Study Commission: Findings of Eleven Years of Activities." *Journal of the Ameri-can Medical Association* 135 (December 1947): 881–84.

Sadove, Max S., James Cross, Harry Higgins, and Manuel J. Segall. "The Recovery Room Expands Its Services." *Modern Hospital* 83 (November 1954): 65–70.

Safar, Paul, T. J. DeKornfield, J. W. Pearson, and J. S. Redding. "The In-tensive Care Unit." *Anesthesia* 16 (July 1961): 275–84.

Sturdavant, Madelyne. "Intensive Nursing Service in Circular and Rectan-gular Units Compared." *Hospitals* 34 (16 July 1960): 46–77.

Thibault, George E., Albert G. Mulley, G. Octo Barnett, Richard L. Gold-stein, Victoria A. Reder, Ellen L. Sherman, and Erik R. Skinner. "Medi-cal Intensive Care: Indications, Interventions, and Outcomes." *New En-gland Journal of Medicine* 302 (24 April 1980): 938–42.

U.S. Army Medical Department. *Surgery in World War II.* Vol. 1, *Thoracic Surgery.* Washington, D.C.: Office of the Surgeon General, Department of the Army, 1963.

U.S. Department of Health and Human Services. National Institutes of Health. *Consensus Conference on Critical Care Medicine.* Washington, D.C.: GPO, 1983.

U.S. Public Health Service. *Coronary Care Units: Specialized Intensive Care Units for Acute Myocardial Infarction Patients,* PHS pub. no. 1250. Wash-ington, D.C.: GPO, 1964.

———. *Facility Designed for Coronary Care.* PHS pub. no. 930-D-19. Wash-ington, D.C.: GPO, 1965.

———. Division of Hospital and Medical Facilities. *Elements of Progressive Patient Care: A Tentative Draft.* PHS pub. no. 59-9467-A. Washington, D.C.: GPO, 1959, microfiche.

W. K. Kellogg Foundation. *The Planning and Operation of an Intensive Care Unit: An Experience Brochure.* Battle Creek, Mich.: W. K. Kellogg Founda-tion, 1961.

Weeks, Lewis E. *The Complete Gamut of Progressive Patient Care in a Commu-nity Hospital.* Battle Creek, Mich.: W. K. Kellogg Foundation, 1966.

Weeks, Lewis E., and John R. Griffith, eds. *Progressive Patient Care: An An-thology.* Ann Arbor: University of Michigan, 1964.

Wilson, Vickie. "From Sentinels to Specialists." *American Journal of Nursing* 90 (3) (October 1990): 32–43.

Woolever, Gloria M. "An Intensive Care Unit." *Nursing Outlook* 6 (Decem-ber 1958): 690–91.

Zalumas, Jacqueline. *Caring in Crisis: An Oral History of Critical Care Nurs-ing.* Philadelphia: University of Pennsylvania Press, 1994.

———. "Critically Ill and Intensively Monitored: Patient, Nurse, and Ma-chine—The Evolution of Critical Care Nursing." Ph.D. diss., Emory University, 1989.

Zschoche, Donna, and Lillian E. Brown. "Intensive Care Nursing: Specialism, Junior Doctoring, or Just Nursing?" *American Journal of Nursing* 69 (November 1969): 2370–74.

General and Medical Technology

American Heart Association. "Closed-Chest Method of Cardiopulmonary Resuscitation." *Circulation* 31 (May 1965); reprinted in *American Journal of Nursing* 65 (May 1965): 105.

American Medical Association. "General Report." In *Commission on the Cost of Medical Care.* Washington, D.C.: American Medical Association, 1964.

American Nurses' Association Committee on Nursing Practice. "Closed Chest Cardiac Resuscitation . . . Professional and Legal Implications for Nurses." *American Journal of Nursing* 62 (May 1962): 94–95.

Baer, Neal. "Cardiopulmonary Resuscitation on Television." *New England Journal of Medicine* 334 (13 June 1996): 1604–5.

Beck, Claude S., Elden C. Weckesser, and Frank M. Barry. "Fatal Heart Attack and Successful Defibrillation." *Journal of the American Medical Association* (2 June 1956): 434–36.

Cowan, Ruth Schwartz. "From Virginia to Virginia Slims: Women and Technology in American Life." *Technology and Culture* 20 (January 1979): 51–63.

———. *More Work for Mother: The Ironies of Household Technology from the Open Hearth to the Microwave.* New York: Basic Books, 1983.

———. *A Social History of American Technology.* New York and Oxford: Oxford University Press, 1997.

Davis, J. Mostyn. "Oxygen Therapy." *Modern Hospital* 79 (November 1952): 98–106.

Diem, S. J., et al. "Cardiopulmonary Resuscitation on Television—Miracles and Misinformation." *New England Journal of Medicine* 334 (13 June 1996): 1578–82.

Grace, William J. "Determinants of Successful Cardiac Resuscitation." In *Proceedings of the Conference on Impact of Coronary Care Unit on Hospital, Medical Practice, and Community,* 14. Arlington, Va.: National Center for Chronic Disease Control, 1966.

Hounshell, David. *From the American System to Mass Production, 1800–1932.* Baltimore: Johns Hopkins University Press, 1984.

Howell, Joel. "The Changing Face of Twentieth-Century American Cardiology." *Annals of Internal Medicine* 105 (1986): 772–82.

———. "Machines' Meanings: British and American Use of Medical Technology, 1890–1930." Ph.D. diss., University of Pennsylvania, 1987.

———. "Soldier's Heart: The Redefinition of Heart Disease and Specialty Formation in Early Twentieth Century Great Britain." *Medical History* (1985): 34–52.

———. *Technology in the Hospital: Transforming Patient Care in the Early Twentieth Century.* Baltimore and London: Johns Hopkins University Press, 1995.

Hughes, Thomas. *A Century of Invention and Technological Enthusiasm.* New York: Penguin Books, 1989.

Keller, Evelyn Fox. *Reflections on Gender and Science*. New Haven, Conn.: Yale University Press, 1985.

Kouwenhoven, William B., James R. Jude, and Guy G. Knickerbocker. "Closed Chest Cardiac Massage." *Journal of the American Medical Association* 173 (9 July 1960): 1064–67.

McDougall, Walter A. . . . *The Heavens and the Earth: A Political History of the Space Age*. New York: Basic Books, 1985.

McGaw, Judith. *Most Wonderful Machine: Mechanization and Social Change in Berkshire Paper Making, 1801–1885*. Princeton, N.J.: Princeton University Press, 1987.

———. "No Passive Victims, No Separate Spheres: A Feminist Perspective on Technology's History." In *In Context: Essays in the History of Technology —Essays in Honor of Melvin Kranzberg*, edited by Stephen H. Cutcliffe and Robert W. Post, 173–74. Easton, Pa.: Lehigh University Press, 1988.

———. "Women and the History of Technology." *Signs* 7 (Summer 1982): 802.

Merchant, Carolyn. *Ecological Revolutions: Nature, Gender, and Science in New England*. Chapel Hill: University of North Carolina Press, 1989.

Morrison, Elting. *Man, Machines and Modern Times*. Cambridge, Mass.: MIT Press, 1966.

National Academy of Sciences. *Medical Technology and the Health Care System: A Study of Equipment Embodied Technology*. Washington, D.C.: National Academy of Science, 1979.

Noble, David R. *America by Design: Science, Technology and the Rise of Corporate Capitalism*. New York: Knopf, 1977.

Reiser, Stanley Joel. "The Machine as Means and End: The Clinical Introduction of the Artificial Heart." In *After Barney Clark: Reflections on the Utah Artificial Heart Program*, edited by Margery W. Shaw, 171–73. Austin: University of Texas Press, 1984.

———. *Medicine and the Reign of Technology*. Cambridge: Cambridge University Press, 1978.

Richards, A. N. "Production of Penicillin in the U.S. (1941–1946)." *Science* 201 (1 February 1964): 441–45.

Russell, Louise B. "The Diffusion of New Hospital Technologies in the United States." *International Journal of Health Services* 6 (1976): 557–80.

———. *Technology in Hospitals: Medical Advances and Their Diffusion*. Washington, D.C.: Brookings Institution, 1979.

Scitovsky, Anne A., and Nelda McCall. *Changes in the Costs of Treatment of Selected Illnesses, 1951, 1964, 1971*. No. 77-2007. Washington, D.C.: Department of Health, Education, and Welfare, 1976.

Showstack, Jonathan, Steven Schroeder, and Michael Matsumoto. "Changes in the Use of Medical Technologies, 1972–1977: A Study of Ten Inpatient Diagnoses." *New England Journal of Medicine* 306 (25 March 1982): 706–12.

Smith, Merritt Roe. *Harpers Ferry Armory and the New Technology: The Challenge of Change*. Ithaca, N.Y.: Cornell University Press, 1977.

Starzl, Thomas E. "Prophylactic Tracheostomy in Aged and Poor Risk

General Surgical Patients." *Journal of the American Medical Association* 169 (14 February 1959): 691–95.

Strauss, Michael. "The Political History of the Artificial Heart." *New England Journal of Medicine* 310 (2 February 1984): 332–36.

Strickland, Stephen P. *Politics, Science and Dread Disease: A Short History of United States Medical Research Policy.* Cambridge, Mass.: Harvard University Press, 1972.

SUPPORT Principle Investigators. "A Controlled Trial to Improve Care for Seriously Ill Hospitalized Patients." *Journal of the American Medical Association* 274 (22–29 November 1995): 1591–98.

Waitzkin, Howard. "A Marxian Interpretation of the Growth and Development of Coronary Care Technology." In *The Sociology of Health and Illness: Critical Perspectives.* 2d. ed., edited by Peter Conrad and Rochelle Kern, 219–31. New York: St. Martins Press, 1986.

Zoll, Paul, Arthur J. Linenthal, Leona R. Norman, Milton H. Paul, and William Gibson. "Treatment of Unexpected Cardiac Arrest by External Electric Stimulation of the Heart." *New England Journal of Medicine* 254 (22 March 1956): 541–46.

Index

Page references followed by "n." or "nn." refer to information in notes; page references in *italics* refer to selected illustrations.